Negotiating Managed Care

A Manual for Clinicians

Negotiating Managed Care

A Manual for Clinicians

Michael A. Fauman, Ph.D., M.D.

Clinical Associate Professor of Psychiatry
University of Michigan School of Medicine
Ann Arbor, Michigan
Medical Director and Vice President for Medical Services
Magellan Behavioral of Michigan, Inc.
Farmington Hills, Michigan

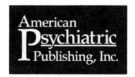

American Psychiatric Publishing, Inc.

Washington, DC
London, England

Note: The authors have worked to ensure that all information in this book concerning drug dosages, schedules, and routes of administration is accurate as of the time of publication and consistent with standards set by the U.S. Food and Drug Administration and the general medical community. As medical research and practice advance, however, therapeutic standards may change. For this reason and because human and mechanical errors sometimes occur, we recommend that readers follow the advice of a physician who is directly involved in their care or the care of a member of their family. A product's current package insert should be consulted for full prescribing and safety information.

Manufactured in the United States of America on acid-free paper
06 05 04 03 02   5 4 3 2 1
First Edition

American Psychiatric Publishing, Inc.
1400 K Street, N.W.
Washington, DC 20005
www.appi.org

Library of Congress Cataloging-in-Publication Data
Fauman, Michael A., 1942-
    Negotiating managed care : a manual for clinicians / Michael A. Fauman.-
- 1st ed.
        p. ; cm.
    Includes bibliographical references and index.
    ISBN 1-58562-042-4 (alk. paper)
    1. Managed care plans (Medical care)--Handbooks, manuals, etc. 2. Negotiation in business--Handbooks, manuals, etc. I. Title.
    [DNLM: 1. Managed Care Programs--organization & administration. 2. Negotiating--methods. 3. Practice Management, Medical--organization & administration. W 130 AA1 F263n 2002]
RA413 .F38 2002
362.1'04258--dc21

                                                    2001053746

British Library Cataloguing in Publication Data
A CIP record is available from the British Library.

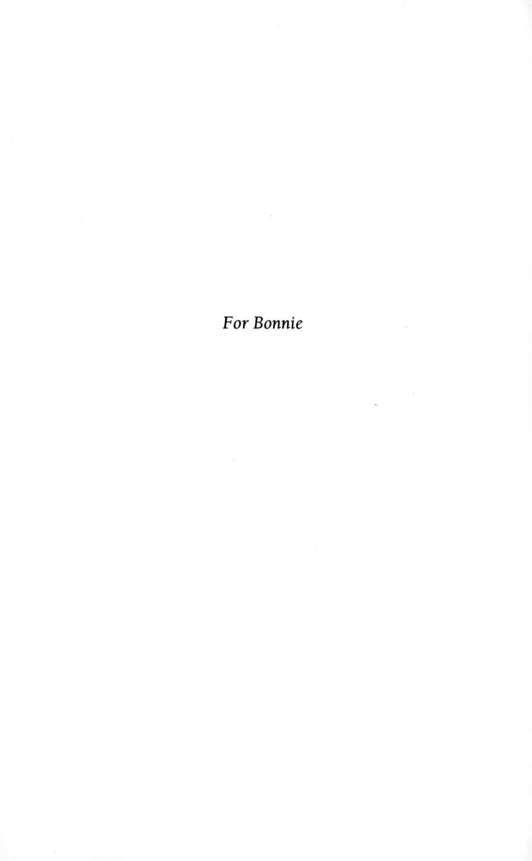

For Bonnie

Contents

CHAPTER 1

Introduction

Acolleague called me the other day to express his anger and frustration at the outcome of a managed care review of one of his cases. The patient was an elderly man with depression and the early symptoms of Alzheimer's disease. He had been living at home with his wife until he became so depressed that he could not get out of bed in the morning. My colleague admitted him to the hospital and immediately began treating him with antidepressant medication. After a week, the man's depressed mood slowly began to abate. At that point, my colleague received a call from a managed care physician, who announced that he was reviewing the case to determine whether the patient needed further hospitalization.

"Why do you think this patient needs further inpatient treatment?" the reviewer asked.

"He's still depressed," my colleague replied.

"Is he suicidal?"

"No, not really."

"Can he be treated in a partial hospital program?"

"He's beginning to respond to the medication and the multidisciplinary therapy we provide on our unit. He can't get the same intensity of treatment in a partial hospital program."

"You can still prescribe the medication in partial, can't you?"

"Yes, but he needs more than that."

"That's a matter of judgment. Unfortunately, he doesn't meet the criteria for inpatient treatment any longer, so we will probably deny additional days."

My colleague was furious as he recounted his conversation with the reviewer. After years of successful practice, he resented being monitored and having his decisions questioned. He complained about the reviewer's seemingly critical and abusive attitude—the suggestion that my colleague was providing unnecessary and wasteful care. "I want to provide the best treatment I can for my patients," he told me. "How can I do that when someone who doesn't even know my patient is allowed to make crucial decisions about his care?"

I could recognize and empathize with his feeling of helplessness, his sense that he no longer had control over his profession. Much of what he said rang true. His story captured in a nutshell the feelings and frustrations of a generation of clinicians—physicians and nonphysicians alike—who have been subjected to managed care reviews.

How did this situation arise? The answer to that question is not complicated: the cost of care increased. As the cost of American health care accelerated at a rate that exceeded inflation in other sectors of the economy, there were increasing calls from business and the government to control these costs. Managed care was the free-enterprise response to these fiscal concerns. It was an attempt to reduce cost by ensuring that patients received only the care they required.

I first encountered the problem of unnecessary care more than 20 years ago, when I ran a psychiatric consultation-liaison service in a large general hospital. One day, the director of the electroencephalography laboratory stopped me in the hall and said, "You aren't ordering any EEGs [electroencephalograms]."

"The patients I see don't need any," I replied.

"You don't know what you may be missing."

"I'll order them when they seem clinically indicated," I responded, with some irritation.

"You don't understand," he said. "You can always justify an EEG, and if we don't get more studies, we'll have to close the lab."

The director's message was clear. He, like I, received weekly accounting summaries from the administration of the hospital listing revenues, expenses, and variances from the budget. Apparently, he needed more business to meet his revenue figures and he was not going to ask whether the requested tests were medically necessary. Medicine has always been as much a business as an intellectual and humanitarian calling. Sometimes, however, the two objectives become confused and business goals become inappropriately couched in the language of medical necessity. Despite the director's protestations, fiscal concerns were influencing his clinical decisions. Yet his behavior also raised questions about the quality and appropriateness of care, given that he was willing to subject patients to the discomfort, inconvenience, and potential danger of a test that they did not need. He had forgotten or ignored both his fiscal and clinical accountability to his patients and profession.

I am sure that most clinicians would be as disturbed as I was about this type of unnecessary care. They are not strangers to fiscal or clinical accountability. Physicians, psychologists, nurses, and social workers have always felt responsible to their patients, their colleagues, their profession, and their society. Why then, do they protest a managed care system that is explicitly designed to curb just such abuses? The answer to this question is no more complicated than the previous one of how managed care arose. Reducing the incidence of unnecessary care can easily become an excuse for denying appropriate care—a process that can generate millions of dollars of extra profit for insurance companies. It all depends on how one defines *necessary* care.

The potential for abuse in a managed care system raises important questions about the review process. Should not accountability work both ways? Are not the reviewers of care obligated to make sure that their decisions are based primarily on patients' clinical needs, rather than the cost of care? There is an apocryphal story that illustrates the concern many clinicians have about this process, the bitterness they feel about having their clinical judgment challenged, and the suspicion they have of reviewers' motives.

One hot summer evening, a young woman brought her boyfriend to a local hospital emergency department. She told the physician that she had walked into her boyfriend's apartment and found him sitting on his bed holding a gun. After some discussion, he admitted to her that he had been thinking of killing himself. The physician spoke with the young man, verified the story, and called the managed care reviewer for approval to admit the patient to the hospital's psychiatric unit. The reviewer questioned him in detail about the patient. "How do you know he actually intended to kill himself?" she asked.

"He said so," the physician replied.

"Was the gun loaded?" she continued.

"I didn't ask."

"Please find out and call me back."

The physician called back a few minutes later to report that the gun had been loaded. There was a short silence.

"Was the hammer cocked?" the reviewer asked.

Here again, the message was clear. The reviewer was engaged in a struggle with the patient's physician. Like a soldier under siege, the reviewer was guarding the ramparts of care against undue intrusion. At the end of this conversation, the emergency physician must have wondered whether he could have said anything that would have convinced the reviewer to approve the patient's admission.

Do either of these two examples represent reasonable ways of providing health care? I do not think so. In the first case, an unnecessary diagnostic test would be approved for purely financial reasons. In the second, the barrier to the provision of care is so high that the service is essentially unattainable. In each case, the patient is ill served. There must be accountability on both sides. The costly resources of care must be preserved, yet they must be made available when truly needed. Currently, the care pendulum swings from one extreme to another, from license to unreasonable restriction.

This book is an attempt to discover a practical and defensible path for the provider between these two extremes. One of the book's fundamental assumptions is that many of the disagreements between reviewers and providers are caused by honest differences in clinical judgment about the severity of a patient's illness and the type of care the patient needs. These disagreements arise because the two groups have both different points of view about how mental health care should be delivered and different amounts of information about the patient. Many people have asked how the clinical judgment of a reviewer, who has not personally interviewed the patient, could possibly be as accurate as that of the provider who treats the patient. That is certainly a valid question. Yet the same question could be asked of a clinical supervisor who never actually sees the patient whose care he or she is supervising. The supervisor relies on the information provided by the patient's therapist. His or her supervision is only as good as the information received. The same is true for a reviewer. There is no question that some reviewers listen for information that will validate their preconceived notions, or make off-the-cuff decisions based on inadequate information. It is to be hoped that they represent a small minority of reviewers. Ethical reviewers consider all the information that a provider presents and base their decisions on that information. The better the provider's presentation, the better the picture the reviewer has of the patient and the more likely it is that he or she will accept the provider's clinical judgment and approve the requested care.

The main goal of this book is to teach mental health practitioners and administrators how reviewers think and how to conceptualize, present, and document clinical care in a manner that greatly increases the likelihood that it will be approved. To achieve this goal, I examine the details of the review process, focus on the potential areas of disagreement between providers and reviewers, and discuss methods of resolving the disagreements. I use brief clinical examples throughout to highlight and discuss each of these areas of disagreement. Important issues discussed are summarized in tables in each chapter. Many of the chapters also contain clinical vignettes that include a clinician's abbreviated presentation of a patient's case followed by a typical reviewer's comments. In each case, the reviewer raises specific questions about the patient's diagnosis, clinical condition, treatment, and response to treatment that he or she expects the clinician to answer. The reviewer's decision depends on the answers to these questions.

Suggested Reading

Barton GM: Private psychiatric practice in an era of managed care. Psychiatr Clin North Am 23:415–426, 2000

Bursztajn HJ, Brodsky A: Captive patients, captive doctors: clinical dilemmas and interventions in caring for patients in managed health care. Gen Hosp Psychiatry 21:239–248, 1999

Croghan TW, Obenchain RL, Crown WE: What does treatment of depression really cost? Health Aff (Millwood) 17:198–208, 1998

Daniels N, Sabin D: The ethics of accountability in managed care reform. Health Aff (Millwood) 17:50–64, 1998

Dubin WR: Can providers and payers collaborate? in Controversies in Managed Mental Health Care. Edited by Lazarus A. Washington, DC, American Psychiatric Press, 1996, pp 291–301

Emanuel EJ, Dubler NN: Preserving the physician–patient relationship in the era of managed care. JAMA 273:323–329, 1995

Friedman LH, Savage GT: Can ethical management and managed care coexist? Health Care Manage Rev 23:56–62, 1998

Glazer WM, Rosenbaum JF: Managed care versus managed money. J Clin Psychiatry 59:62–66, 1998

Green SA: Is managed care ethical? Gen Hosp Psychiatry 21:256–259, 1999

Kassirer JP: Managed care and the morality of the marketplace. N Engl J Med 333:50–52, 1995

Lazarus JA, Sharfstein SS: Ethics in managed care. Psychiatr Clin North Am 23:269–284, 2000

Marquis MS, Long SH: Trends in managed care and managed competition, 1993–1997. Health Aff (Millwood) 18:75–88, 1999

Rodwin MA: Conflicts in managed care. N Engl J Med 332:604–607, 1995

Sabin JE: What our students teach us about managing care ethically. Psychiatr Serv 49:879–881, 1998

Swartz K, Brennan TA: Integrated health care, capitated payment, and quality: the role of regulation. Ann Intern Med 124:442–448, 1996

CHAPTER 2

Clinical Monitoring, Standards, and Liability

The stated goal of managed care is to ensure that every patient's treatment is appropriate and cost-efficient. The main process that managed care uses to achieve this goal is clinical monitoring, which includes discussions with providers and reviews of documentation. The information gathered through monitoring is compared with a set of specific standards and used to make decisions to approve or deny payment for clinical services. Managed care organizations are protected by federal law from malpractice suits that might result from these decisions, although these protections are coming under increasing attack in the courts. The more you understand about the details of this review process, the better you will be able to use the process to gain what you want for your patients and protect yourself from medical liability.

Clinical Monitoring

There are two main types of clinical monitoring. *Concurrent monitoring* occurs while care is being provided. It includes an initial precertification stage that occurs before treatment begins. *Retrospective monitoring,* also called *utilization review,* occurs after care has been delivered (Table 2–1). Most clinical monitoring done by managed care companies since the early 1990s has been concurrent. There are two reasons for this. First, in concurrent monitoring, reviewers are involved in the provision of each episode of care from the be-

---

Table 2-1. Types of clinical monitoring

Precertification review
Performed before treatment begins, to determine whether the patient meets
criteria for a specific type of care such as hospitalization.

Concurrent review
Performed during treatment, to determine whether the patient requires continuing treatment.

Retrospective review
Performed after completion of treatment, to determine whether the patient's
illness justified the type of treatment he or she received. Retrospective reviews
are always based on clinical documentation.

---

ginning. This allows them to decide whether care is appropriate and necessary before it has been rendered and to provide immediate feedback to the
clinician. It is less useful, from a clinical or fiscal standpoint, to decide that
care is inappropriate after it has been delivered. That only leads to endless
negotiations and litigation among reviewers, insurance companies, patients,
and clinicians. If, in the final determination, the care is deemed unnecessary,
it has been wasted. Second, the information management technology necessary to implement concurrent monitoring was not readily available until the
early 1990s. Many years before the introduction of concurrent monitoring,
clinicians and administrators concerned about the cost of care were well
aware of the advantages of such a process. They were hampered by the need
for enormous computing resources to gather, store, and retrieve the necessary patient information.

A few rough calculations will demonstrate the scope of these resources.
Let us assume that an insurance company provides coverage for 1 million
subscribers and measures the utilization of services by calculating the number of hospital or inpatient days used, each year, per 1,000 subscribers. *Days
per thousand* is the standard measure for utilization in the insurance industry. Let us assume further that the utilization for this group of subscribers is
25 days per 1,000. This means that each year the insurance company pays
for 25,000 hospital days. If the average length of stay is 5 days, there will be
5,000 admissions during the year. On average, a reviewer will speak to the
provider or a facility representative approximately three times during a patient's hospitalization. The initial contact will be for *precertification*—that is,
to obtain prior approval for the admission. After admission, a reviewer will

talk with the facility representative or provider every 2 or 3 days until the patient is discharged. Therefore, the reviewers will have approximately 15,000 discussions each year, or 60 each workday. Each of these discussions must be documented, often in great detail. Furthermore, because a facility representative may call at any time and speak to different reviewers, a patient's record must be instantly available to every reviewer. This combination of computing power and accessibility—the capacity to store large amounts of data and make them instantly available to many people over a computer network—simply did not exist before the mid-1980s. Thus, the current revolutionary changes in medical practice, including concurrent monitoring, could not have occurred without these developments.

Given the superiority of concurrent monitoring, why is retrospective monitoring still performed? One main reason is that some cases never undergo concurrent monitoring. The provider and the hospital representative may not bother to call for precertification, or concurrent monitoring may not have been implemented in their area. In these situations, the only way to review the appropriateness of care is by retrospective monitoring. Second, and more important, there is often some question about the validity of the information obtained through the concurrent process. Consider how concurrent monitoring is performed. A provider or hospital representative calls the reviewer, describes the patient's clinical signs and symptoms, and asks for approval for treatment. The reviewer makes a decision on the basis of this oral report. Subsequent reviews and requests for additional treatment are made in a similar fashion. The only information the reviewer has is that provided by the caller.

The reviewer may question the validity of the information he or she receives from the caller. In many cases, the caller requesting approval for care has no direct clinical contact with the patient. He or she may be a hospital employee without much clinical training who is simply reading portions of the patient's medical record to the outside reviewer. The patient's clinical picture can look very different, depending on the specific information the caller has available and chooses to read from the record. If, for example, the caller reports that the patient has made threats against her mother but the caller has no details about the threats or information on the circumstances under which they occurred, the reviewer may not be willing to approve the hospitalization concurrently and may ask the facility representative to send the medical chart for retrospective review after the patient is discharged.

A different problem can occur if the caller is the patient's physician or therapist. In this case, the provider may consciously or unconsciously distort the information in a manner that makes the patient's condition seem worse than it actually is, thereby convincing the reviewer to approve the requested care. One can imagine a situation in which a patient says, "I could kill my mother" and the patient's provider tells the reviewer that his patient threatened to kill her mother. The provider may actually be convinced that the patient is dangerous although the latter made only a qualified statement, saying what she *could* do, rather than what she *would* do. Reviewers routinely request a patient's medical chart if they suspect there is a discrepancy between what they have been told and the patient's actual clinical status and treatment. Some insurance companies randomly request medical charts as a way of statistically checking the validity of the concurrent process and the appropriateness of care.

The main advantage of a retrospective review for inpatient work is that it provides a broad base of information about the patient's condition, because the medical chart contains observations and comments by all members of the mental health staff—nurses, social workers, psychologists, activity therapists, occupational therapists, and physicians—who have evaluated and treated the patient. Many times this information verifies what the hospital representative, physician, or therapist reported over the telephone. In other situations, the various observations, made by different or even the same clinicians, reveal discrepancies. Some of these may be subtle, but others may be quite blatant. These discrepancies represent one of the many elements of uncertainty that are a normal part of the clinical process and its review. Many occur even when the care has been excellent. Only a small number are the result of overt attempts at deception. The appropriateness of clinical oversight depends on how these uncertainties are judged and resolved.

Although the breadth of clinical information available through retrospective review offers an advantage over concurrent monitoring, the process also has some potential problems. The most obvious of these is clinical hindsight. Suppose, for example, a patient is admitted to the hospital because of overt suicidal ideation. The patient remains in the hospital for 5 days, even though she denies suicidal ideation by the third day, because the psychiatrist wants to be certain that she will not harm herself. By the time the retrospective review takes place, long after the patient has been discharged, the reviewer knows whether the patient has made a suicide attempt. If she has not, the reviewer might decide to deny the last 2 days of the patient's hospitalization—perhaps reasoning that the extra days were unnecessary, given that the patient ultimately did not harm herself. This is obviously not a rational basis for denying days of care. A sensible reviewer will put himself or herself in the position of the provider treating the patient. The provider has no way of knowing in advance how the patient will do after discharge. He or she must make a clinical decision about discharge based on clinical experience and the patient's history. Depending on the provider's confidence in his or her clinical judgment and the particular circumstances of the case, the provider might want additional time to be certain that the decision is correct. The question is, how much extra time is necessary? No matter what the answer, the reviewer cannot ethically base his or her decision on prior knowledge of the patient's outcome. To do so would be an abuse of the monitoring process.

The problem of clinical hindsight is one of the most frustrating aspects of a retrospective review for providers, because providers feel that the reviewer is second-guessing their clinical decisions without actually seeing or speaking with the patient. For example, the reviewer may have seen documentation that a patient denied having suicidal ideation, but because the reviewer did not observe the patient do so, he or she is not aware of the quality of the denial. Did the patient deny having suicidal ideation tentatively, offhandedly, cynically, ironically, or with resignation, or was her statement convincing? A clinician's treatment decisions often rest on such subtle observations. Moreover, because the reviewer is not responsible for the patient, the reviewer can make any decision he or she wishes without fear of the consequences. Suppose the psychiatrist had discharged the patient as soon as she denied having suicidal ideations and the patient then killed herself. The reviewer could retrospectively approve the patient's hospitalization without any questions about the psychiatrist's clinical judgment.

The contention of some clinicians that retrospective reviews are, by their very nature, biased against them has some validity. Yet there are other providers who have considerably less trouble than their colleagues with such reviews. Why is this so? Part of the answer lies in the manner in which clinicians document their clinical observations and treatment decisions. The clinicians who have less trouble with reviewers are those who are able to convey in their notes enough detailed clinical information about the patient, and the quality of the patient's interactions, to convince the reviewer that their decisions are correct.

In theory, a retrospective review can have both an educational and a deterrent value. It is educational when it offers useful feedback to facilities about their standards of care and to providers about the quality of their clinical documentation. It is a deterrent when it prods facilities and providers to correct any problems in care and documentation so that they can continue to be reimbursed for the services they provide. However, these educational and deterrent values are present only if the retrospective review is timely and contains detailed information about the nature of any problems that have been discovered. If the review is conducted several months after the patient's discharge, memories of the clinical details will fade and the process will seem irrelevant. If the reviewer's critique is superficial or vague, it will seem more like harassment than potentially useful feedback.

Clinical Standards Defined

Clinical monitoring requires some standard that defines the appropriateness of care and against which the care in question is measured. There are several other common names for standards, including criteria, guidelines, and yardsticks. They are all essentially the same thing—a set of rules that can be used to make a decision or define a category. Some standards are very precise; others are less definite and subject to a wide range of interpretation. The best-known example of a mental health standard is the *Diagnostic and Statistical Manual of Mental Disorders,* now in the fourth edition with revised text (DSM-IV-TR), published by the American Psychiatric Association. Other important clinical standards include medical necessity criteria, substance abuse treatment criteria, and clinical practice guidelines. All of these standards play an important role in monitoring the quality and efficiency of care provided to individuals with psychiatric disorders.

DSM-IV-TR is a collection of criteria sets for the diagnosis of psychiatric disorders. The criteria for each disorder specify those signs and symptoms that must be present or absent to verify a diagnosis. The resulting diagnosis allows practitioners to accurately communicate important information about a patient's illness in a clinical shorthand. In a sense, DSM-IV-TR provides a set of rules that can be used to reproducibly differentiate two illnesses. If, for example, I tell you that a patient has a dysthymic disorder, you immediately have a picture of a person who has had a persistent depressed mood and other defined symptoms for a specific length of time. You can differentiate that picture from the one associated with another diagnosis such as major depressive disorder. The diagnostic criteria may also tell us something about the etiology of the patient's illness, its natural history, and its response to treatment.

Medical necessity criteria differ from diagnostic criteria in that their focus is on the need for medical care rather than the signs and symptoms necessary to make a specific diagnosis. Although most medical necessity criteria involve at least a tentative diagnosis, more importance is placed on the presence or absence of symptoms such as self-destructive behavior, delusions, or hallucinations that, by themselves, would not meet the criteria for a specific diagnosis. The central concept of most medical necessity criteria is the *level of care* determination (Table 2–2). Levels of care can be thought of as points

Table 2-2. Mental health and substance abuse treatment levels of care

Hospitalization
Hospitalization permits provision of intense 24-hour psychiatric, nursing, and other multidisciplinary services for patients with acute psychiatric disorders. Hospitalization is the highest level of care.

Residential care
Residential programs provide multidisciplinary services for patients with less acute disorders who do not require intense psychiatric treatment but who do require 24-hour supervised care.

Partial hospital care
Partial hospital programs provide intense psychiatric, nursing, and other multidisciplinary services for patients who require care for less than 24 hours a day. Patients usually attend for a minimum of 4 hours a day, several days a week.

Intensive outpatient treatment
Intensive outpatient programs provide multidisciplinary therapy and counseling for patients who need treatment several hours a week.

Traditional outpatient treatment
Traditional outpatient programs provide various forms of individual and group psychotherapy for patients who require treatment once a week or less. Traditional outpatient treatment is the lowest level of care.

on a scale that ranks the various types of clinical management according to the resources necessary to provide that management. Determining level of care also involves determining which clinical problems are best addressed by each type of management. In that sense, levels of care make up an economic as well as a clinical scale. Determination of level of care is an attempt to provide a patient with safe, appropriate, and effective treatment that makes the most efficient use of medical resources.

Outpatient treatment is the lowest level of care in most medical necessity criteria. The term *lowest* in this case refers to the amount of clinical resources necessary to deliver adequate outpatient care, not to the quality or appropriateness of the care. Outpatient treatment is the lowest level of care because it can be provided by a single clinician in his or her office. Outpatient care can be stratified according to the efficient use of resources by considering the intensity and duration of treatment sessions and the training of the therapist. An hour of outpatient treatment provided once a week by someone with a bachelor's degree in counseling costs less than the same treatment provided over the same length of time by a master's-level social worker, a psychologist, or a psychiatrist. However, some people have argued that this approach is not necessarily more cost-efficient in the long run. It does little good to use a lower-paid therapist to treat a patient if that therapist does not have the expertise to do the job efficiently and successfully. It is always easy to find someone with less expertise who charges less. The challenge is to match the patient's problems with a therapist who has the appropriate training to treat those problems.

As the level of care increases, the amount of resources expended on treatment increases as well. In intensive outpatient therapy, a patient is seen several times a week rather than once. In a partial hospital program, the patient is treated by several therapists for at least half the day. At the highest level of care, hospitalization, a full range of multidisciplinary services is offered and the cost of care increases accordingly. The difference in cost is striking. Whereas outpatient treatment costs as little as $50 a week, inpatient treatment can cost 50–100 times as much. This enormous cost differential is a strong motivating factor to assign patients to the lowest level of care consistent with good treatment. Inpatient care is generally reserved for the most severe mental health problems, usually defined as problems resulting in an imminent threat of a patient's doing serious harm to self or others or problems resulting in the danger of a patient's being seriously harmed because the patient cannot adequately care for himself or herself. The latter might involve situations in which the patient's clinical state is deteriorating despite appropriate outpatient management or situations in which the patient's response to medications requires close monitoring.

Clinical practice guidelines go one step beyond diagnostic criteria and medical necessity criteria. They specify the type of care that a patient with a specific diagnosis or set of symptoms should receive. In many cases, clinical practice guidelines incorporate elements of the diagnostic and medical necessity criteria. A clinical practice guideline for the treatment of major depressive disorder, for example, will generally state that the patient must meet DSM-IV-TR criteria for the diagnosis of major depressive disorder. In addition, it will usually specify those clinical parameters that necessitate inpatient versus outpatient care. Clinical practice guidelines are far more detailed than medical necessity criteria. The major reason for this is that there are a number of different, although equally acceptable, ways of treating the same psychiatric disorder. Major depressive disorder, for example, can be treated with insight-oriented psychotherapy, cognitive-behavioral therapy, antidepressant medication, or a combination of these treatments. Some research suggests that mild to moderate major depressive disorders may also be successfully treated using a self-administered computer program.

A simple example may help clarify the role of the three standards. Consider a 26-year-old man who is brought to the emergency department of a local hospital by his father, who claims that the patient, normally a friendly, cooperative, and hard-working man, has undergone a dramatic change in his personality over the last several months. In the past month, the patient, who lives with his father, has become increasingly secretive and irritable and has developed a number of odd behaviors. Most noticeable of these is his habit of sitting alone in the kitchen shaking his head and mumbling. On the occasions when his father asked him what he was doing, the patient became angry and stalked out of the house. These episodes of isolative behavior alternated with periods when the patient angrily complained about his boss. His father finally brought him to the hospital when the patient stated that he would have to "settle the score" with his boss by himself.

In the hospital, the patient eventually admitted to the psychiatrist that he heard a voice telling him to settle the score with his boss, but he would not be specific about what that meant. The psychiatrist, using DSM-IV-TR, made a provisional diagnosis of schizophrenia, paranoid type. Once the diagnosis was made, the psychiatrist had to decide what level of care the patient required. The deciding factor was not so much the presence of auditory hallucinations but the nature of those hallucinations and how the patient responded to them. Many patients have auditory hallucinations, even after optimal treatment, but can ignore them and carry on with their lives. The voices occupy a corner of their minds, producing a low background hum. For others, however, the voices occupy center stage and cannot be ignored. The most pernicious of these hallucinations are the ones in which voices command the patient to perform some act of violence. In the case described, the psychiatrist interpreted the patient's auditory hallucinations as a threat that he might seriously harm his boss. On the basis of this interpretation, the psychiatrist decided that the patient met the medical necessity criteria for inpatient hospitalization.

The psychiatrist's final decision concerned the patient's treatment. Many clinical practice guidelines would suggest that the patient be treated with one of the newer atypical antipsychotic medications, such as olanzapine, quetiapine, risperidone, or clozapine, given that he was apparently suffering from an initial, acute psychotic episode. Once the acute symptoms were under control, the patient would need reality-oriented supportive therapy, education about his illness, access to support groups, and assistance in obtaining necessary resources and services.

The Need for Clinical Standards

Why are clinical standards necessary? Why do reviewers not simply accept the decisions made by credentialed practitioners? There are two main reasons for clinical standards. First, there are many ways to diagnose and treat mental illness, and not all of these are appropriate or effective. Second, practitioners—even credentialed clinicians who have completed high-quality training programs and are board certified in their specialties—vary widely in their abilities and competence. When there are no standards, clinical anarchy exists, with little control over the consistency or quality of the treatment provided by different practitioners. The ability to distinguish between appropriate and inappropriate diagnoses and treatments disappears, and irrational theories and modes of treatment proliferate.

Nonetheless, not all clinicians believe that established clinical standards are useful. That fact was highlighted for me one afternoon while I was teaching a seminar on outpatient psychiatry. I had just emphasized the importance of making a diagnosis before beginning treatment when one of my senior residents challenged me. "Why do I need to make a diagnosis?" he asked. "If a patient is depressed, I'll start him on an antidepressant medication. If that doesn't work, I'll add lithium or an anticonvulsant. If that doesn't work, I'll add an antipsychotic or a benzodiazepine. Eventually something will work. How will a specific diagnosis change that?"

My resident was making two somewhat provocative points. First, he was arguing that treatment should be based on a patient's symptoms, not a diagnosis. If a patient is depressed, he concluded, why not simply treat the patient's depressed mood and forget about trying to make a diagnosis of a specific depressive disorder? Second, he was suggesting that the pharmacological treatment of depression was a rather unscientific process. From his point of view, the process consisted of trying one medication after another, in an almost random fashion, until some combination worked. Having reviewed hundreds of clinical cases, I am convinced that this type of clinical reasoning occurs more frequently than one would expect or wish in general psychiatric practice.

Were my resident's observations and conclusions correct? I do not think so. He was arguing that all depressive illnesses are the same with respect to their symptoms and responses to treatment. In his mind, a depressed mood completely defined the illness. Experienced clinicians would disagree. They know that there are several varieties of depression and that these varieties are distinguished by differences in etiology, the type and intensity of symptoms, the duration and frequency of episodes, and response to treatment. There are even patients with a depressive illness who are not aware of feeling depressed. These varieties of depression, characterized by specific clusters of signs and symptoms, constitute distinct syndromes or disorders that can be reliably identified by different clinicians using specific diagnostic criteria.

Investigations designed to assess the effectiveness of new treatments for depression routinely use such diagnostic criteria to identify groups of patients with the same depressive disorder. If they did not, the positive response of patients with one depressive disorder might be masked by the lack of response by those with a second disorder. Strictly speaking, then, the results of such studies are applicable only to the specific diagnostic categories of illness that were targeted in the investigation. The finding of one study that lamotrigine is very effective in the treatment of bipolar I depression is not automatically applicable to the treatment of a major depressive disorder or a dysthymic disorder. The effectiveness of lamotrigine in the treatment of those disorders can be determined only by further research. The use of such research to guide treatment is the basis for the contemporary movement of evidence-based medicine. Eventually, results of these studies will be incorporated into clinical practice guidelines.

My resident's approach to prescribing medication was also a problem. It assumed that every depressed patient requires medication, despite repeated evidence that many patients can be effectively treated by some form of psychotherapy. Furthermore, my resident would expose his patients to several unnecessary drugs, each with its own spectrum of side effects, and would potentially prolong their suffering, because many of the drugs he mentioned require a minimum trial of 2 weeks or more before their effectiveness or lack of effectiveness can be determined. Finally, his approach was very inefficient. Each medication that was tried and found ineffective substantially increased the cost of his patient's treatment. One main goal of clinical practice guidelines is to reduce such unnecessary treatment by using the results of well-controlled research studies and expert opinion to guide practitioners toward the therapeutic approach that is most likely to be effective. This entire system starts with an accurate diagnosis. The diagnosis provides a stable base and common denominator for comparison among patients, studies, treatments, and practitioners. A similar argument can be made for some medical necessity criteria and clinical practice guidelines.

Interpreting Clinical Standards

There are many appropriate and effective ways to diagnose and treat mental illness. A reexamination of the case of the young schizophrenic patient discussed earlier can help to illustrate this. He was brought to the hospital and there admitted hearing a voice telling him to "settle the score" with his boss. The psychiatrist interpreted the patient's statement as a threat to seriously harm his boss and, following the medical necessity criteria, hospitalized the patient. Was this an appropriate decision? Perhaps, but a second psychiatrist might have given the same patient some antipsychotic medication and referred him to an outpatient clinic.

Given the patient's symptoms, how could a second psychiatrist justify not hospitalizing him? The answer to that question depends on how the second clinician interpreted the patient's symptoms and the medical necessity criteria. Suppose she interpreted the phrase *settle the score* as an indication that the patient was angry at his boss—that he might sue the boss, start screaming at him, or sabotage his work—and not as evidence that he would try to seriously harm the man. Now one has two diametrically opposed yet equally defensible interpretations of the patient's symptoms and the medical necessity criteria. The first psychiatrist prefers to interpret the criteria liberally. To him, any threat should be considered a threat of serious harm unless proven otherwise. The second psychiatrist makes a more conservative interpretation. She must have evidence beyond a few simple words to conclude that a patient will seriously harm someone. Who is correct? At the moment the decision is made, it is impossible to say who is correct. Furthermore, even if the patient actually tried to harm his boss, this would not constitute proof that another patient reporting similar symptoms would be likely to seriously harm someone. Although medical necessity criteria, diagnostic criteria, and clinical practice guidelines serve different purposes, they have this quality in common: they are subject to different, yet equally defensible, interpretations by different clinicians.

Suppose one changes the example and assumes that the second psychiatrist was reviewing the case to approve or deny the patient's admission to the hospital. Now the provider must defend his clinical assessment and treatment decision to the reviewer. The situation is no longer an academic disagreement between colleagues, the possible subject of an interesting clinical conference. The patient's immediate care depends on the reviewer's decision. This hypothetical encounter raises several important questions. How should the standards—the medical necessity criteria in this case—be interpreted? Was the first clinician's decision correct? What information does he need to support his decision? How should he present that information? Stated more succinctly, the major question is the following: How can the frequent differences of professional opinion between clinicians and reviewers be resolved in a manner that provides the patient with the safest, most effective, and most efficient care possible? That question is the main focus of this book.

Many clinicians would argue that such a resolution is difficult, if not impossible, because the actual goal of most reviewers is to reduce cost, not ensure that a patient receives appropriate care. There is no question that this is true of some reviewers. They serve a gatekeeper role in the health care system, unreasonably denying higher-level care to all but the sickest patients. In such cases, the only recourse may be litigation or appeal through insurance regulatory agencies. Yet many other reviewers are ethical, clinically experienced, current in their knowledge, amenable to reason, and willing to compromise. They listen closely to the provider's clinical evaluation of the patient and base their judgment on several points: Is the presentation organized? Does it contain sufficient details to convince the reviewer that the provider understands the patient? Is it consistent with other information the reviewer has about the patient? Finally, does it make clinical sense and follow accepted clinical practice guidelines?

In sum, the clinical review can best be characterized as a negotiation between provider and reviewer. The provider tries to convince the reviewer that the patient is sick enough to require the requested level of care. The reviewer tries to make certain that the provider is presenting an accurate description of the patient and that the request for service is justified based on a reasonable interpretation of the clinical standards. Currently, this is an unequal negotiation. The provider is at a disadvantage because he or she has only the power of persuasion, whereas the reviewer has the power to approve or deny the request for clinical service. Many practitioners think that it is unfair to expect them to spend their time trying to learn how to negotiate with a reviewer. They maintain that the time would be much better spent providing clinical service or perfecting the tools of their trade. Theoretically, that may be true. Who, however, cannot benefit from feedback and critical review? Reviews may not always be pleasant, but they force clinicians to examine what they are doing and make corrections where necessary. Many other practitioners do not believe that they should have to justify how they treat their patients to a reviewer. Unfortunately, that is not a realistic expectation in the current age of managed care. Providers will be far more successful if they learn how to identify, gather, organize, interpret, and communicate relevant clinical information in a consistent, reliable, and convincing manner.

Clinical Liability

Conscientious providers occasionally tell reviewers who have denied a request for care that the reviewers will be held legally responsible for the repercussions of their decisions. That is currently incorrect. Managed care is possible because managed care companies and their reviewers are not held legally liable for patients who suffer from denials of care. Unfair as it may seem, the patient's provider is still the one who is almost always liable for an adverse outcome. The courts generally find that a provider's clinical obligations to a patient supersede financial considerations. Therefore, a provider cannot use a reviewer's denial as an excuse to immediately stop treating a patient whom he or she or other competent clinicians believe requires care.

Managed care organizations and their reviewers are protected from medical liability suits by the Employee Retirement Income Security Act (ERISA), which was enacted by Congress in 1974 to control pension and health benefit plans. Although states traditionally regulate medical care and malpractice litigation, ERISA preempts state medical liability laws so that they can no longer be enforced in court. At the same time, ERISA does not contain federal medical regulation or liability provisions to replace the state laws. Members of Congress are currently trying to address this issue with the proposed patients' bill of rights. The intent is to restore some local control over health benefit plans that come under the ERISA umbrella. It is not yet clear what impact this would have on managed care reviews, but it would almost certainly increase the utilization and short-term cost of health care.

The ERISA preemption is also under attack in the courts. A distinction has been made between litigation over the quantity versus the quality of care. The former has been interpreted by most courts as completely preempted by ERISA, whereas the latter is not. This means that there may be an increasing number of suits regarding the quality and safety of medical care, rather than the amount of care approved or denied. This distinction is one of several ongoing attempts to narrow the ERISA preemption and extend managed care's liability.

Given the current state of health care liability under ERISA, how should you respond to denials of care? You are obviously not obligated to treat patients for free when a reviewer denies care. When making a decision to discharge a patient after such a denial, however, you should be guided primarily by your clinical assessment of the patient, just as you would for any other treatment decision. Suppose, for example, you hospitalize a patient with suicidal ideation and intent. After the patient has been in the hospital for 3 days, the reviewer denies further inpatient care. What should you do? If you believe that the patient's suicidal ideation and intent are significantly resolved, and you requested additional inpatient days only to consolidate the patient's clinical gains, you might reasonably decide to discharge the patient. However, if you believe that the patient is still suicidal, you have an obligation to keep the patient in the hospital, even if the reviewer disagrees with your assessment. If you discharge the patient under those circumstances and the patient commits suicide, you, not the reviewer, may be held legally liable.

The situation is very different if the patient's illness is not life threatening. Suppose you are treating a nonsuicidal patient for depression in your office and the reviewer denies your request for additional treatment sessions. It may be that the patient no longer has benefits or that the reviewer believes that the patient does not meet the medical necessity criteria for additional treatment. What are your options if you believe that the patient requires further treatment? First, appeal the denial. If the appeal is not successful, you can ask the patient to pay out of pocket for the sessions. If the patient is unwilling or unable to pay for treatment, you can refer the patient to a local community mental health center. If you do refer the patient to another therapist, make sure that you provide clinical coverage until the patient is seen by the new provider. Often a reviewer will allow two or three transition sessions to enable you to transfer the patient without a hiatus in treatment.

No matter how unfair you believe the reviewer's decision might be, you should always act in the patient's best interest. Do not let your frustration with the managed care company and its reviewer inappropriately influence your clinical decisions. Make sure you document in the patient's record everything you do and why you do it. This is especially important when the reviewer denies care, because you want to make certain there is evidence that you appropriately considered the patient's clinical status when you made your decisions.

Suggested Reading

American Psychiatric Association: Diagnostic and Statistical Manual of Mental Disorders, 4th Edition, Text Revision. Washington, DC, American Psychiatric Association, 2000

American Society of Addiction Medicine: ASAM Patient Placement Criteria. Chevy Chase, MD, American Society of Addiction Medicine, 1992

Appelbaum PS: Pegram v. Herdrich: the Supreme Court passes the buck on managed care. Psychiatr Serv 51:1225–1226, 2000

Bartels SJ, Levine KJ, Shea D: Community-based long-term care for older persons with severe and persistent mental illness in an era of managed care. Psychiatr Serv 50:1189–1197, 1999

Bloche MG: U.S. health care after Pegram: betrayal at the bedside. Health Aff (Millwood) 19:224–227, 2000

Calabrese JR, Bowden CL, Sachs GS, et al: A double-blind placebo-controlled study of lamotrigine monotherapy in outpatients with bipolar I depression. J Clin Psychiatry 60:79–88, 1999

Davidson BN: Managing behavioral health care: an employer's perspective. J Clin Psychiatry 59:9–12, 1998

Fleishman M: What is psychiatric "medical necessity"? Psychiatr Serv 51:711–712, 2000

Fuchs VR: No pain, no gain. JAMA 269:631–633, 1993

Geddes J: Asking structured and focused clinical questions: essential first step of evidence-based practice. Evidence-Based Mental Health 2:35–36, 1999

Hetznecker W: Are practice guidelines useful in managed care? in Controversies in Managed Mental Health Care. Edited by Lazarus A. Washington, DC, American Psychiatric Press, 1996, pp 41–54

Hrehor KR, Renick O: The legal challenge to ERISA preemptions. Empl Benefits J 26:25–29, 2001

Koike A, Klap R, Unutzer J: Utilization management in a large managed behavioral health organization. Psychiatr Serv 51:621–626, 2000

Kramer TL, Daniels AS, Zieman GI, et al: Psychiatric practice variations in the diagnosis and treatment of major depression. Psychiatr Serv 51:336–340, 2000

Kuder AU, Kuntz MB: Who decides what is medically necessary? in Controversies in Managed Mental Health Care. Edited by Lazarus A. Washington, DC, American Psychiatric Press, 1996, pp 159–177

Mariner WK: What recourse? liability for managed-care decisions and the Employee Retirement Income Security Act. N Engl J Med 343:592–596, 2000

McAuliffe BE: The changing world of HMO liability under ERISA. J Leg Med 22:77–106, 2001

Mechanic D: Managed care and the imperative for a new professional ethic. Health Aff (Millwood) 19:100–111, 2000

Mihalik G, Scherer M: Fundamental mechanisms of managed behavioral health care. J Health Care Finance 24:1–15, 1998

Miller KA, Miller EK: Lexicon of managed care concepts and terms, in Making Sense of Managed Care. Edited by Miller KA, Miller EK. San Francisco, CA, Jossey-Bass, 1997, pp 1–15

Moffic HS: Training psychiatric residents in managed care. Psychiatr Clin North Am 23:451–459, 2000

Moskowitz EH: Clinical responsibility and legal liability in managed care. J Am Geriatr Soc 46:373–377, 1998

Nonacs R, Cohen LS: Postpartum mood disorders: diagnosis and treatment guidelines. J Clin Psychiatry 59:34–40, 1998

Osgood-Hynes DJ, Greist JH, Marks IM: Self-administered psychotherapy for depression using a telephone-accessed computer system plus booklets: an open U.S.-U.K. study. J Clin Psychiatry 59:358–365, 1998

Rosenquist P, Colenda CC, Briggs J, et al: Using case vignettes to train clinicians and utilization reviewers to make level-of-care decisions. Psychiatr Serv 51:1363–1365, 2000

Rosenthal MB, Geraty RD, Frank RG, et al: Psychiatric provider practice management companies: adding value to behavioral health care? Psychiatr Serv 50:1011–1013, 1999

Rosoff AJ: Breach of fiduciary duty lawsuits against MCOs. What's left after Pegram v. Herdrich? J Leg Med 22:55–75, 2001

Sabin JE: What our students teach us about managing care ethically. Psychiatr Serv 49:879–881, 1998

Sabin JE, Daniels N: Public-sector managed behavioral health care, II: contracting for Medicaid services—the Massachusetts experience. Psychiatr Serv 50:39–41, 1999

Sisk JE: How are health care organizations using clinical guidelines? Health Aff (Millwood) 17:91–109, 1998

Stone A: Paradigms, pre-emptions, and stages: understanding the transformation of American psychiatry by managed care. Int J Law Psychiatry 18:353–387, 1995

Stone AA: Managed care, liability, and ERISA. Psychiatr Clin North Am 22:17–29, 1999

Sturm R: Tracking changes in behavioral health services: how have carve-outs changed care? J Behav Health Serv Res 26:360–371, 1999

Terry K: Where's managed care headed? Med Econ 77:244–260, 2000

Treatment of schizophrenia 1999. The Expert Consensus Guideline Series. J Clin Psychiatry 60 (suppl 11):3–80, 1999

Trueman DL: Managed care liability today: laws, cases, theories, and current issues. Journal of Health Law 33:191–262, 2000

CHAPTER 3

Presenting Your Case to a Reviewer

Much of your success in the current mental health care system depends on your ability to convince reviewers to approve the care you think will best serve your patients. That approval, in turn, depends on your ability to present and argue your patient's case effectively. Presenting a clinical case is a skill that most practitioners learn in training. However, making a clinical presentation to a professional care reviewer from a managed care or insurance company is somewhat different from presenting the same case to a teacher or colleague. You expect helpful critiques from teachers and useful suggestions and support from colleagues. Care reviewers, on the other hand, are usually strangers who are more interested in determining whether you can justify your treatment decisions than in providing you with useful suggestions and support. The review itself, usually conducted over the telephone, is more formal and distant than a presentation to a colleague. You may feel judged and criticized during the discussion, even if the reviewer does not make any overt critical statements. Despite these differences, however, many of the principles of clinical presentation that you were taught in your professional training can be applied—albeit with some change in tactics—to the current process of clinical review and accountability.

Professional reviewers are skeptics—some even say cynics—who start with the bias that most patients probably do not need the level or intensity of care the practitioner is requesting. That bias—based on their experience reviewing hundreds of cases—may or may not be appropriate, but it is a fact of life in the current environment of clinical accountability. Your goal is to provide the reviewer with sufficient relevant information to convince him or her that your patient does require the level of care you are requesting. This is not an impossible task, but it does require more thought and planning than you have been accustomed to devote to the process in the past. Everything you do in the review should be directed toward presenting an effective argument in favor of your treatment plan. Anything that detracts from your presentation decreases the likelihood that your request will be approved. In this chapter, I provide you with guidelines that you can use to make more effective presentations to reviewers (Tables 3–1 and 3–2).

Table 3-1.   General presentation guidelines

- Assume that the reviewer is ethical unless you have direct evidence to the contrary.

- Reviewers are not clinical supervisors. Do not expect helpful critiques, suggestions, or support from them.

- Give the reviewer sufficient information to convince him or her that your patient needs the care you request.

- Be prepared to defend your clinical decisions.

- Revise your presentation style if your requests are frequently denied, even if you think you present cases well.

I have said that if you cannot defend your clinical decisions, the reviewer will deny care. Unfortunately, this does not mean that the reviewer will always approve care when you present a cogent and convincing argument. Some unethical reviewers will deny care no matter what the case. No amount of preparation on your part will convince such reviewers to approve care, because their goal is to cut costs without regard for clinical consequences. I will discuss how to deal with this type of reviewer later in the book. A great many other reviewers, however, are ethical, willing to listen to you present your case, and willing to judge the case as objectively as possible.

If you are like most clinicians, you are convinced that you already present your cases adequately. If reviewers are approving a high proportion of your requests for patient care, your assumption is probably correct. If, however, you spend inordinate amounts of time arguing with reviewers or find that they frequently deny your requests, it might be helpful to review some of the guidelines in this book.

Table 3-2. Successful presentation techniques

- Think of every review as a negotiation. Be willing to compromise with the reviewer.

- Act as the patient's advocate. Do not ask the patient or his or her family to protest the reviewer's decision.

- Put the patient's welfare first in every decision you make. Do not let your anger at the review process influence your clinical decisions.

- Be open to feedback from the reviewer even if you do not agree with him or her. Be ready to reexamine your management of the patient's case.

- Try to establish a friendly working relationship with the reviewer so that he or she will learn to trust your judgment.

- When you disagree with a reviewer, state your objections clearly and politely and then appeal the reviewer's decision.

- Present a realistic assessment of your patient's clinical status. Do not exaggerate his or her signs or symptoms.

- Be available to talk to the reviewer.

- Document your discussion with the reviewer in the patient's medical record.

Negotiate, Negotiate, Negotiate

Several years ago, the rules for running a clinical practice were clearly defined and nonnegotiable. Practitioners stated their fees and determined how, and for how long, they would treat patients, and insurance companies complied with their demands. All that has changed. To be successful today, a practitioner must be a good negotiator as well as a good clinician. The type of bargaining that is common in business and government has finally reached the day-to-day practice of medicine, social work, psychology, and nursing. I am not talking about bargaining just for office space, supplies, and staff. The art of bargaining also applies to the clinical review process. Every review is a negotiation (Table 3–2).

Many practitioners, especially those who have been in practice a long time, are uncomfortable negotiating services with a reviewer. They still expect their clinical decisions to be accepted without question. This is not surprising given that negotiation was never part of the curriculum of any mental health clinical training program in the United States. As a provider, you decide how to treat your patient based on your training and on what you have found clinically effective. You may have developed a small number of routine treatment protocols that seem to work for you. The reviewer, however, knows that there are often many effective treatments for the same disorder and that these treatments may differ significantly in cost. He or she is looking for a treatment that is both effective and efficient.

How can you convince a reviewer to approve your request? First, you must accept that negotiating on behalf of your patient is not a professional loss of face; it is simply a new aspect of the job of being a clinician. Be realistic when you negotiate. Do not expect the reviewer to meet all your demands. Decide on an alternative or fall-back position before you begin the discussion. Because you cannot always receive approval for the services you initially request, you must bargain for some portion of those services or lose them all to a denial. Negotiating is not as implausible or degrading as it may seem. Most reviewers do not like to deny services. They would rather arrive at a negotiated settlement with the provider in which they feel they have trimmed the unnecessary services yet allowed the provider enough time and resources to treat the patient successfully. Reviewers will become increasingly more willing to negotiate as patients gain the right to sue health maintenance organizations and managed care companies for denying care.

The most important thing to remember about the process of negotiation is that you must have reasonable arguments to back up your requests for care. It is not sufficient to assume the reviewer will automatically understand that your demands are justifiable. Part of the negotiation process is helping the reviewer understand why your request is reasonable. The more effectively you present your case, the more likely you are to have your request approved. What I am talking about, therefore, above and beyond the clinical issues of the case, are the tactics of negotiation. In this chapter, I discuss the various components of the clinical negotiation process and make recommendations that you can use to improve your success in the process. More specifically, I discuss how you should orally present your case to a reviewer to achieve the highest likelihood of approval.

When you negotiate, your initial demands cannot be so unrealistic that the reviewer will immediately reject them. In practical terms, this means that if you are a psychiatrist who wishes to admit a psychotic patient to the hospital, you should not begin by asking the reviewer to approve 10 days of care. Because few reviewers will approve 10 days in an initial request, the demand will be seen as naive, unrealistic, or provocative. At the same time, do not be so intimidated that you ask for only 2 or 3 days. Present the details of your case to the reviewer and ask for approval for, say, 5 days of hospitalization. Make sure you can defend why you need 5 days instead of 3 or 4. That establishes a reasonable base negotiating position.

Manage Your Anger

You probably resent having to seek approval from a reviewer before treating your patients. It seems inherently unfair that someone can come between you and your patients. Yet reviews are a fact of professional life in an age of clinical accountability. The important thing to remember is that you should not let your anger interfere with the review or with your ability to help your patient (Table 3–2).

It may be tempting, when you feel frustrated with a specific review or reviewer, to enlist the patient or the patient's family in the protest against the reviewer's decision. Some physicians virtually turn over responsibility for an appeal to the patient and family. One angry psychiatrist told his patient's family that he had done everything he could to get the patient's care approved, and he instructed the family to call the medical director of the insurance program to protest the reviewer's denial of care. If you were this psychiatrist, you might feel some momentary satisfaction after making these statements—satisfaction that the reviewer would finally experience some of the same pressures placed on you by the patient, family, and hospital administration—but what you said to the family in your anger would not help your patient much. You are the patient's best advocate. If you give up that responsibility, the patient will suffer. Although pressure from family, political figures, and other influential people can sometimes overturn a reviewer's decision, the long-term effect of such intervention will be to damage your relationship with the reviewer. In the end, the reviewer will be far less willing to give you the benefit of the doubt in future cases. Furthermore, you can use this tactic only a few times before the insurance company officials and hospital administrators begin to wonder why you have so many problems managing your cases. This will only stimulate them to look in more detail at your patient management. Eventually, patients and their families will also resent that you are asking them to perform a function that is legitimately part of your job. Although you may feel some immediate satisfaction at turning the tables on the reviewer, in the end you and your patients will suffer.

Do not let your indignation at the review process make you do things that are against your patient's best interests. In one case, a psychotic patient who was involuntarily admitted to the hospital refused to take medication. The court hearing for commitment to a psychiatric institution was delayed for 3 weeks. During those 3 weeks, the reviewer discussed the case several times with the patient's psychiatrist and approved hospital days, despite the fact that the patient could not be treated with medication until the court commitment proceedings had been completed. Five days after the patient was committed, the reviewer called the provider to discuss the patient's progress. She discovered that the provider had started treatment with a sub-therapeutic dose of antipsychotic medication a few days earlier and had not increased the dose. When she asked the provider why he had not increased the dose, he responded that he was trying to get the patient's cooperation. The reviewer pointed out that the patient had been committed because he was unable or unwilling to be cooperative with the treatment and that the court order allowed the provider to administer the dose he thought appropriate. The psychiatrist responded that he did not want the reviewer telling him how to practice. The next day he discharged the patient.

You might argue that the reviewer had no right to pressure the psychiatrist to increase the patient's medication. The reviewer saw the situation differently. She was charged with ensuring that the patient was treated in a manner that was efficient and that complied with the prevailing standards of care in the community. That was the context in which she was trying to understand the psychiatrist's reason for increasing the dose of medication so slowly. Despite her misgivings, she continued to recommend to the insurance company that further days of care be approved. The psychiatrist, on the other hand, resented her continued monitoring. This resentment, more than the patient's clinical condition, seemed to be the immediate motivating factor in his decision to discharge the patient.

You may also be tempted to deal with your frustration during a review by becoming angry at the reviewer. Some providers use this as a general tactic. They become indignant and combative during each review. A few even insult the reviewer, openly questioning his or her ethics and clinical competence. This is not surprising, given the fact that the reviewer is the most visible symbol of the clinical oversight system, and he or she often bears the brunt of the practitioner's anger. The reviewer, of course, is only trying to do his or her job. He or she will not automatically be empathic to your frustrations. Although you may feel some relief in venting your anger, getting angry will not help you get what you want. It may in fact have just the opposite effect. Reviewers do not have the option of getting angry in return. Instead, they try to avoid such practitioners. They will try to limit the amount of time they spend talking with an angry provider—thereby limiting the amount of information that the provider can present about the patient.

Reviewers also become increasingly suspicious of practitioners who always become angry during a review, especially when the practitioners constantly switch from a discussion of the patient to a tirade against managed care. If you do this, the reviewer may interpret your change of topic as an attempt to avoid talking about the patient. He or she may conclude that you do not know much about the patient or cannot effectively manage the patient's illness. Therefore, the reviewer is more likely to deny your request and ask to have the medical chart sent in for review after the patient is discharged. This subjects you to even more detailed scrutiny and increases the likelihood that the services you provide will be denied in retrospect.

The best tactic to use in a review is to be reasonable and avoid getting overtly angry at the reviewer. Be open to feedback. This does not mean that you must agree with the reviewer's decision. It does mean that you should be willing to reexamine what you are doing. Maybe you can change how you manage the case. Can you, for example, complete the patient's treatment in a shorter period? Ask yourself whether you have overlooked something. Ask yourself whether you are angry because the reviewer's decision is inappropriate or because you resent having to participate in a review.

Because there are a relatively small number of reviewers, compared with the number of providers, it is likely that you will work with the same reviewer many times. Try to establish a friendly working relationship with the reviewer instead of wasting your time getting angry at him or her. Once the reviewer learns to trust your judgment, he or she will be more likely to go along with your treatment plan and suggestions in the future. It is not as difficult to establish such a working relationship as it might seem. Most reviewers do not enjoy denying care. Many are looking for a reason to grant your request. If a reviewer has worked with you before and can trust your judgment, he or she will feel justified in approving care even if the particular details of the case would not normally convince the reviewer to do so. The best way to establish this trust is to be honest with the reviewer, listen to his or her concerns, and respond to them directly.

Do Not Exaggerate

There is often a temptation, when you present a case to a reviewer, to exaggerate the patient's signs and symptoms to make the patient seem sicker than he or she is so that the reviewer will recommend additional days of hospitalization (Table 3–2). Exaggeration of a patient's clinical status can take many forms. Sometimes this exaggeration is innocent. The provider's initial evaluation of the patient may lead the provider to believe that the patient is sicker than he or she really is. In subsequent encounters, the practitioner moderates his or her opinion of the severity of the patient's illness. This type of exaggeration stems directly from the uncertainty that is a normal part of every clinical evaluation.

A few practitioners, however, go beyond exaggeration and openly lie about their patients' symptoms. Most clinicians who practice conscious deception justify it by arguing that they are protecting their patients from insurance company reviewers who are less interested in the patients' care than in cutting costs. It is understandable that clinicians wish to be an advocate for their patients. It is also understandable that clinicians may consider the review process unfair. Nevertheless, when a provider lies, he or she is placed in a precarious ethical and negotiating position. If the reviewer asks for additional details, the provider often finds himself or herself caught in a web of deception. Furthermore, the reviewer has too many channels of information that he or she can use to cross-check information presented by the provider to be deceived for long. Eventually, inconsistencies become apparent, especially if the patient's medical chart is reviewed after his or her discharge.

One psychiatrist, for example, reported that his patient was acutely suicidal and that she had stated that she would kill herself if she were not hospitalized immediately. A subsequent examination of the medical record showed that the patient denied suicidal ideation to other clinical staff members during admission and repeatedly thereafter. Another psychiatrist told the reviewer that he needed to keep a patient hospitalized for several more days because there was evidence that the patient might be having seizures and an adverse reaction to his medication. The reviewer asked a case manager to follow the patient's progress. She spoke with the utilization review manager at the hospital, who read her the patient's medical record over the telephone. There was no documentation in the medical record suggesting that the patient had a seizure disorder or that he was having an adverse reaction to his medication. It soon became apparent that the provider was telling the reviewer whatever was necessary to keep the patient in the hospital.

Providers who exaggerate or lie about their patient's symptoms eventually make their professional lives more difficult. Once the deception becomes apparent, the reviewer will no longer trust the provider. He or she is more likely to demand additional clinical details and be more skeptical in the future. Furthermore, because reviewers often talk about their experiences among themselves, they will soon all be alert to the deceptive practices of an individual provider.

Make Yourself Available

Arranging a time for two clinicians to speak together can be more complicated than the actual negotiations that take place during the review. The process frequently degenerates into a form of telephone tag, in which the reviewer calls the provider and leaves a message, only to have the provider return the call at a time when the reviewer is unavailable. This process can continue for several days after the patient's treatment has begun. Unfortunately, it is your responsibility as a provider to speak with the reviewer in a timely fashion. You might believe that if you are unable to discuss the case with the reviewer until after the patient has been in the hospital for 2 or 3 days, the reviewer will be forced to recommend approval for the care the patient has already received. Unfortunately, this is not correct. Reviewers will generally not recommend approval for those days unless the patient meets the criteria for care.

Every review organization has a policy for dealing with providers who do not respond to a reviewer's call. In most cases, the reviewer is required to make a set number of calls over a certain period. Once these calls have been made, the case is automatically denied for lack of contact. Therefore, it is to your advantage as a provider to respond to the reviewer's call as quickly as possible. This is especially important if there is some likelihood that the reviewer will recommend that the care you wish to provide for your patient not be approved.

One psychiatrist made it a habit to engage in long periods of telephone tag with the reviewer. He instructed his secretary to intercept every call from a reviewer and take a message. Then he returned the call in the evening, after normal business hours. The reviewer responded to this tactic by calling the psychiatrist at home in the evening. He soon began to respond in a more timely fashion. Another psychiatrist, when called by a reviewer to discuss a case, routinely requested to discuss the case the following day, stating that he did not have the patient's record available. The next day, when the reviewer called, the psychiatrist informed him that the patient had been discharged. The discharge did not satisfy the reviewer, because he realized that it was the physician's way of avoiding talking about the patient. When this happened repeatedly, the reviewer concluded that the physician either was trying to keep his patients in the hospital as long as he could without being challenged or else did not know what to do with his patients. In either case, the reviewer's response was the opposite of what the physician desired. Rather than paying less attention to the physician, the reviewer began paying more attention.

The best way to deal with a reviewer's call is to respond as quickly as possible and negotiate for your patient's care. If your secretary handles your calls, have him or her tell the reviewer that you will be available at a specific time to discuss the case. Make sure you are available. Alternatively, have your secretary ask the reviewer when it would be convenient for you to call back. The reviewer will generally respond to your courtesy by doing everything he or she can to be fair.

Reviewers expect to experience some delays in contacting providers. They usually are also clinicians with busy schedules and understand that it is difficult to return calls in the limited time between patient appointments. If, however, they detect a pattern of repeated delays, they become suspicious that the provider is being manipulative and are far less likely to give the provider the benefit of the doubt in the future. Again, as when practitioners are deceptive, the provider's cases are scrutinized more closely. The reviewer assumes that if the provider is evading a review, he or she may also be hiding other things that should not be approved.

Denials and Appeals

No matter how carefully you prepare your presentation, there will be times when the reviewer will not recommend that care be approved. How should you respond when the reviewer denies your request for care? First, review your request again, in your own mind. Ask yourself whether you really need the additional time for the patient. Can you can work more efficiently and finish the patient's treatment within the allotted time? Try to be honest with yourself. Do not let your annoyance with the process interfere with your ability to make a rational decision about the patient's care. If you are convinced that your request is justifiable, ask the reviewer if he or she would feel comfortable approving some part of the request, perhaps half the number of days. Explain that you will do your best to treat the patient as efficiently as possible. This is the type of situation in which it is useful to have a good relationship with the reviewer. If you have been honest with the reviewer in the past, he or she will probably give you the leeway to treat the patient as you see fit.

If the reviewer remains unconvinced by your arguments, ask for an appeal. Every clinical review organization has an appeal process. You will have a stronger case if you appeal the decision immediately, while the patient is still receiving care. Make sure you document your conversation with the first reviewer. Present your case to the second reviewer as if you had not presented it to the first reviewer. Be certain that you include all the details. Try not to let your irritation at the first review influence the tone and manner in which you present to the second reviewer. In many cases, the clinical argument that did not work during the initial review will convince the second reviewer to recommend approval of some days of care.

Before you present an appeal, make sure you have read the medical necessity criteria and understand the specific clinical information that the reviewer needs to make a decision. Most companies will provide you with copies of their medical necessity criteria. Identify which criteria you believe the patient fulfills and how the patient fulfills them. If the second reviewer also recommends that further care be denied, ask him or her to explain the reasons for this decision. If the reviewer will not explain, document his or her refusal. If the first appeal is unsuccessful, write a letter to the review organization and the insurance company (if they are separate entities) detailing your specific concerns. Request a further review of the case, essentially a second appeal. This may be an internal review or an external review with an entirely separate review organization.

Unreasonable Reviewers

Whenever a reviewer refuses to recommend that care be approved, ask him or her to explain the basis for this decision in some detail. Reviewers commonly ask clinicians to provide clinical details about their cases. The reviewer's decision depends on these details. Therefore, it is appropriate to ask the reviewer to explain his or her decision in some detail. You will be able to determine the reviewer's motivation very quickly, depending on how he or she responds to your question. Some reviewers will be happy to discuss their decision-making process with you and to help you understand it for future cases. Others may become irritated at your request.

There are two main types of reviewers. The first type is reasonable, willing to discuss the case with an open mind, and amenable to negotiation. Everything I have said so far assumes that you, as the practitioner, are speaking to such a reviewer. The second type of reviewer is not so reasonable. If, after honestly trying to work with a reviewer, you become convinced that he or she is acting unprofessionally, note the specifics of the reviewer's behavior and write a formal letter of protest to the managed care or insurance company. In the better companies, reviewers are given feedback on how providers perceive them. If there are too many protests from practitioners, or if the medical director sees a pattern in the protests, he or she will intervene and provide additional training for the reviewer. In some cases, the medical director will stop using the reviewer.

Some unreasonable reviewers, however, work for companies that habitually underbid to win contracts. Because the low bid provides a very slim margin, reviewers who work for these companies are instructed to deny care whenever possible, to save money. When the typical inpatient stay was 20 or 25 days, the length of inpatient care could be decreased relatively easily. These days, when the average length of stay is 5–8 days, it is more difficult to justify denying days of care. In fact, the role of the reasonable reviewer is not to further reduce the number of hospital days but to ensure that the length of hospitalization does not creep up again to previous unacceptable levels. For companies that work on a slim margin, however, cutting even an additional half-day of care may make the difference between a profit and a loss. Their reviewers are much more aggressive than those from rival companies who have not underbid their contracts and who do not feel the need to squeeze every last dollar out of the care system.

Your problem, as the practitioner, is to decide how to respond to an unreasonable reviewer who does not appear to have much concern for the patient's welfare. It will not help to argue with such a reviewer, because you have different goals. Neither will it help to become angry or make threats. Reviewers who deny many requests for care are accustomed to having providers become angry with them. They may in such situations feel even more justified recommending that care be denied, because they interpret the anger as a sign that the provider cannot rationally argue his or her case. How, then, should you proceed? First, provide the care that the patient needs, even if it is not approved. Then appeal the case as described earlier in "Denials and Appeals." If you are unsuccessful after exhausting all the levels of appeal stipulated in the contract with the review company, you must carry your protest further. The best way to do this is to write a detailed letter, describing the circumstances of the case, to the state insurance commission or agency that regulates insurance companies. When the appeal reaches this level, the patient and his or her family will probably also have to request that the state agency review the case. This will often lead to a hearing before the agency, during which you, your patient, and your patient's family will have the chance to confront representatives of the insurance and review companies directly. During the hearing, the insurance commissioner may simply listen to the arguments or may try to arbitrate between the parties to reach a compromise settlement. The final decision is usually issued several weeks later.

Carrying an appeal to the level of the state insurance commission takes a considerable amount of time and preparation. It is not something you would want to do to protest the denial of 2–3 days of care. Most such appeals involve 30 or more days of care, representing thousands of dollars of denied payment. Insurance companies and review organizations realize that you will not spend the necessary time to protest an individual denial of 2 or 3 days of care. If, however, you and your colleagues discover a particularly egregious series of denials from a single reviewer or company, it might be worth your time to present them as a group to the state insurance agency.

CHAPTER 4

Presenting an Inpatient Case

One of the most common complaints I hear from reviewers is that practitioners do not provide them with sufficient, relevant clinical information to allow them to make decisions. This is particularly true of requests for hospitalization. To approve a hospitalization, a reviewer must compare the patient's signs and symptoms with a set of medical necessity criteria to determine whether the criteria are fulfilled. The reviewer is unable to do this without detailed clinical information about the patient's condition. Although it may seem unreasonable, a simple statement that a patient is psychotic or suicidal is not sufficiently detailed to fulfill the medical necessity criteria. The reviewer will ask for more details because he or she is held accountable for his or her decision and must document the clinical particulars that support it.

Remember, every review is a negotiation. Your strategy in this negotiation should be to gain control of the review with a skillful presentation. To do this, you need to anticipate what the reviewer requires and supply that information before he or she asks for it. If you do not, the reviewer will begin asking detailed questions about your patient. Once this happens, you have lost control of the review. One question will lead to another, and the reviewer may stray into areas you do not want to discuss. Furthermore, the very fact that he or she had to ask detailed questions will make it look as though you do not know how to manage your patient's treatment.

Four Questions to Answer

The best way to provide the information that the reviewer needs is to organize it as a response to the four questions listed in Table 4–1. These four

Table 4–1.   Four questions to answer in every inpatient care review

- Why does the patient need to be hospitalized now?

- What are you trying to accomplish with the hospitalization and how will you know when you have accomplished it?

- How will you treat the patient?

- What are you planning to do with the patient after discharge?

questions can be applied to every level of clinical care. Each question can be divided into more specific questions, depending on the patient's symptoms and the level of care you think the patient requires. I discuss inpatient care in this chapter because hospitalization is the highest, most costly level of care and therefore the one monitored most closely by reviewers. Partial hospital is discussed in a subsequent chapter.

Why does the patient need to be hospitalized now?   The first question is the most important. You must quickly establish why your patient needs hospitalization. Medical necessity criteria for inpatient hospitalization are fairly similar (Table 4–2). Their focus is on the severity of the patient's illness and the intensity of clinical service necessary to treat the illness. They stipulate that the patient must be a danger to self or others or be so unable to care for himself or herself that intensive psychiatric and nursing services are required on a 24-hour basis. Therefore, you must be certain that the clinical details you present to the reviewer clearly establish that the patient meets these criteria. The reviewer will not accept your clinical judgment of the case unless you provide the detailed information that allowed you to reach that conclusion (see Case 4–1). You should recognize that the level of clinical detail you consider appropriate may not be considered appropriate by the reviewer. You may, for example, consider it sufficient to tell the reviewer that your patient is psychotic and delusional or that he or she has suicidal ideation. Those statements, however, do not provide sufficient information for the reviewer to determine whether the patient meets the medical necessity criteria for 24-hour acute inpatient care. He or she will want more specific details.

Table 4-2. Generic medical necessity criteria for psychiatric hospitalization

---

- The patient must have a DSM-IV-TR psychiatric disorder that can be expected to benefit from inpatient treatment.

- There must be clear evidence that the patient is a danger to self or others, unable to care for self, or experiencing significant complications of treatment.

- The patient requires intense psychiatric and nursing care on a 24-hour basis.

- The patient cannot be safely assessed or treated at a lower level of care such as in a partial hospital or outpatient program.

Case 4–1: "He is very anxious"

Clinical presentation: A psychiatrist called for approval to admit to the hospital, directly from his office, a 49-year-old man with anxiety. When asked to describe the patient's clinical condition in more detail, she replied, with some irritation, "He is very anxious. That's all."

Reviewer's response: What makes this patient's anxiety so severe that it cannot be treated in an outpatient setting? What is meant by *very anxious*? What are the patient's associated signs and symptoms? How does the anxiety affect his life? Does he have a severe panic disorder? Is there an underlying psychosis? Has the patient undergone prior unsuccessful outpatient trials of medication or cognitive-behavioral therapy?

I said earlier that each of the four main questions can be divided into several more detailed questions. If a reviewer is not satisfied with a statement that a patient has suicidal or homicidal ideation, what additional information might he or she need to justify admission (see Case 4–2)? Think back to your professional training. Would your clinical supervisor be satisfied with a presentation that consisted only of the statement that your patient has suicidal ideation? The supervisor would probably ask you to tell him or her more about the case. He or she would want to know details about the nature of the suicidal ideation. Does the patient have fleeting thoughts of suicide, or does he or she think of suicide continuously? Has the patient made a suicide attempt? Does the patient intend to act on his or her thoughts and try to commit suicide? Has the patient recently been hospitalized for the same problem? If so, how many times? Is the patient currently in outpatient treatment with the provider? Your supervisor would also expect you to be sensitive to the finer clinical details of the case. The supervisor might point out that there is a subtle but important difference between asking a patient how he or she would try to kill himself or herself and asking whether the patient actually intends to kill himself or herself and how the patient intends to do it. Many people muse about how they could kill themselves. Far fewer actually intend to kill themselves.

Case 4–2: "Cindy tried to buy a gun!"

Clinical presentation: Cindy is a 36-year-old woman whose family had her involuntarily admitted to the hospital for treatment of a hypomanic episode and homicidal ideation after she discontinued her lithium therapy. She was intrusive and irritable and had rapid speech. Her family reported that she had "tried to buy a gun to shoot her husband." She had threatened to kill her husband twice before but had not acted on the threats. The facility requested approval for admission.

Reviewer's response: The staff needs to provide more detailed information about the patient's clinical state, especially her homicidal ideation and intent. Did Cindy actually go out to buy the gun or simply threaten to do so? At what stage in the process was she detained? Had she ever acted violently toward her husband or anyone else? How likely was she to do anything violent? Could lithium therapy safely be restarted on an outpatient basis? Could family members have exaggerated Cindy's threat to kill her husband because they felt overwhelmed by her behavior and could not think of any other way to obtain treatment for her?

When you present your patient's symptoms, do not assume that the reviewer will automatically draw the correct conclusions about the severity of those symptoms and the likelihood that they will place the patient in significant jeopardy. Reviewers tend to minimize a patient's symptoms unless there is convincing information to the contrary. It is not sufficient, for example, to report that a patient required admission to the hospital because she had problems with memory and was confused. You must indicate why those symptoms place the patient in significant danger. One argument might be that the patient's memory loss and confusion were of recent onset and might reflect a serious medical problem that can be evaluated and treated only in the hospital. Another argument might be that the patient is so confused that she is endangering herself by wandering into heavy traffic, driving her car in a dangerous manner, or forgetting to turn off the burners on her stove.

What are you trying to accomplish with the hospitalization? Once you have explained why your patient needs care, you must answer the second question and describe what you are trying to accomplish by hospitalizing the patient. What goals have you set for the patient's treatment? How will you know when the goals you have set for the patient's treatment have been met? Here again, you must be specific. It is not sufficient to speak in generalities such as "I want to treat the patient's psychosis." That is like telling a travel agent that you want to take a trip without saying where you want to go or how you want to get there. The details are just as important in clinical care as they are in other areas of life. It may seem implicit, when you treat a patient with antidepressant medication, that your treatment goals will be met when the patient is less depressed. However, that may not necessarily be the case. Not all patients with a major depressive disorder have depression as their main symptom. A good reviewer will not automatically assume that a reduction in depression is the appropriate treatment goal for this patient. You need to be specific about what outcome you expect to see if the treatment is successful. In the case of a confused, elderly woman with a major depressive disorder, you might expect a significant reduction in her confusion as she responds to medication. Suppose, on the other hand, you are treating a young man with a major depressive disorder whose main symptom is a pervasive feeling of worthlessness. Presumably, you would expect him to develop a more positive sense of self-worth if treatment was successful. Both patients are depressed, but in each case a different symptom predominates. Although these distinctions seem like elementary clinical practice, they are often ignored by providers when they present cases to reviewers. Unfortunately, reviewers sometimes interpret this lack of clinical specificity as an example of the provider's evasiveness.

How will you treat the patient? Once you have established that the patient meets the criteria for immediate hospitalization, you must answer the third question and tell the reviewer how you plan to treat the patient. Present a brief but detailed treatment plan. If you decide to use medication to control the disorganized thinking and behavior of a patient with schizophrenia, discuss specific doses. You might say, "I am going to start the patient on 4 mg of risperidone per day and gradually increase the dose to 6–8 mg, until his symptoms are under control or he develops significant side effects." If you want to admit a severely depressed patient who failed to respond to multiple antidepressant medications as an outpatient, summarize the prior treatment before describing your new treatment plan. You might tell the reviewer, "I tried this patient on 60 mg of fluoxetine, switched her to 150 mg of venlafaxine when the fluoxetine did not work, augmented the venlafaxine with 10 mg of olanzapine, and gradually added 200 mg of lamotrigine a day. None of these worked. I want to hospitalize her to try a course of electroconvulsive therapy."

Make sure that the treatment you propose is consistent with current standards of care. When asked why he had prescribed 25 mg of thioridazine to a patient with a major depressive disorder with psychotic features, one psychiatrist replied, "In my experience, Mellaril is a good antidepressant." The reviewer had no way of knowing what the practitioner had actually experienced, but he did know that Mellaril (thioridazine) is not generally considered an antidepressant medication and that the dose the psychiatrist prescribed was probably too low to treat the psychosis effectively. Therefore, as far as the reviewer was concerned, the treatment was not appropriate because it did not meet accepted standards of practice as described in contemporary clinical practice guidelines such as those published by the American Psychiatric Association. The psychiatrist might have justified his choice of the type and amount of medication had he stated that he was using it to treat the patient's psychosis, rather than his depression, and had he explained that the patient was very sensitive to the medication or had experienced side effects with higher doses.

A good reviewer will not, or should not, challenge a practitioner's clinical judgment. He or she may, however, ask for some verification that the mode of treatment chosen by the practitioner is supported by evidence in the professional literature. Reviewers are not necessarily aware of all the latest treatment modalities, so the request for verification may represent a desire for self-education as well as an attempt to give the practitioner the benefit of the doubt. A few years ago, one of our reviewers reported that a psychiatrist was prescribing lamotrigine, a drug he had not heard of, to a patient with a bipolar disorder. The reviewer had not seen the early reports in the literature that lamotrigine might be useful in the treatment of this disorder. He had some concerns about the relevance of this treatment until he saw the reports. If you are going to use a treatment that is new, experimental, or unusual, you can prevent such misunderstandings by gathering citations from the professional literature that support your treatment decision.

What will you do with the patient after discharge?   The final question you must answer in the review is what you are planning to do with the patient after his or her discharge. In the past, providers had the luxury of waiting several days before starting discharge planning. That is no longer feasible. You cannot think of the patient's illness in piecemeal fashion. You must conceptualize all the stages of the patient's treatment as components of a unified episode of illness. Once you decide to hospitalize the patient, you will have a finite amount of time before you must discharge him or her. Therefore, you should be thinking about the discharge plans the moment you make the decision to hospitalize. Be specific about these plans when you present them to the reviewer. If problems develop during the patient's treatment, revise the discharge plans accordingly. If you begin talking about discharge plans during the initial review, the reviewer will know that you are doing your best to be as efficient as possible in taking care of the patient. Here again, the details are important. Do not tell the reviewer merely that you are going to send the patient to an aftercare program when he or she is discharged. Be more specific. State which program you will send the patient to, and indicate whether you have had a conversation with the program staff about the patient.

If you will refer the patient to an outpatient therapist after discharge from the hospital, talk with that therapist when you admit the patient and make sure you have a clear understanding of the circumstances under which the patient will be accepted for treatment after discharge. This will minimize problems with referral that occur when the patient is ready for discharge. Reviewers will generally not approve additional days of care for patients who are clinically stable but waiting for discharge plans to be finalized. Therefore, if you begin to aggressively work on the patient's discharge at the time he or she is admitted, you are more likely to have all the days of care you request approved.

In the most successful presentations, the practitioner answers all four questions so effectively that the reviewer has few remaining questions of his or her own. It takes experience and practice to present a concise, cogent, and effective summary of a patient's illness. The most common mistake that practitioners make is to ramble in their presentations and include irrelevant clinical details that have nothing to do with the reviewer's decision. Here is an example of an effective presentation that is limited to the relevant clinical information:

> The patient is a 33-year-old woman who has become increasingly depressed and withdrawn over the last 3 weeks. During that time, she has appeared confused and unable to perform her normal daily functions including attending to her hygiene, cleaning the house, and performing adequately in her job as a sales clerk in a large department store. All of these are significant changes from her normal state. A few days ago, the patient developed a psychotic delusion that an odor was emanating from her that disgusted everyone around her. She also began to hear voices telling her that she was a wicked person and must destroy herself. The day before admission, she tried to kill herself by slashing her wrists with a rusty pair of

garden shears. Although the cuts were superficial, the psychiatrist who examined her thought she was a significant danger to herself and admitted her to our psychiatric service.

I think this patient has a major depressive disorder with psychotic features. I plan to treat the psychosis with olanzapine, starting with 2 mg twice a day and increasing the dose until the psychotic symptoms are under control. I will treat the depression with sertraline, starting at 50 mg/day and increasing the dose to 200 mg/day during the first week if there are no side effects.

When a Patient Is Not Responding

Suppose you have a patient who, despite your best efforts, is not responding to treatment. How should you respond to the reviewer's questions? Some providers ask the reviewer for suggestions. Generally, this is not a good idea. Consider the contradictions in what you are saying when you ask for suggestions. On the one hand, you are asking the reviewer to approve additional days of care. On the other hand, you are telling the reviewer that you do not know what to do with those days. Some reviewers may be all too willing to tell you how to treat your patient, although you may not like their suggestions. Most reputable reviewers, however, will refuse to offer treatment advice because this could be interpreted as an attempt to take charge of the patient's care. Doing so might make them subject to malpractice litigation. A reasonable reviewer will bypass the potential liability inherent in a request for assistance by engaging you in a dialogue that will help you decide how to proceed with the patient's treatment. He or she might, for example, ask a series of questions to help you explore various treatment options and their consequences. If that does not work, the reviewer may suggest that you consult with a colleague. In either case, the reviewer will be left with the impression that you do not know how to manage the patient. Remember, the reviewer is not acting as your colleague. His or her job is to evaluate the patient's need for care, not help provide care.

Let us assume that you have a patient who meets the diagnostic criteria for a major depressive disorder. The patient has been in the hospital for 3 weeks and has not improved despite trials of two antidepressant medications. She is deeply depressed, anorexic, hopeless, and helpless and has significant psychomotor retardation and thoughts of killing herself. Let us also assume that the reviewer is pressing you to do something for the patient. How should you reply? The key to an effective response is a cogent treatment plan that anticipates the potential problems in treatment and describes how you will respond to them. You might state, for example, "I am going to keep this patient on the same medication for 1 more week to see if she will respond. During that time I am going to increase the medication to the maximum appropriate dose." The reviewer is likely to ask what you will do if the patient remains unresponsive to the medication. An appropriate reply might be "If the patient does not respond to this medication within 1 week, I will consider using electroconvulsive therapy. I plan to begin the patient's workup for electroconvulsive therapy today."

When your patient is not responding to treatment, the best way to answer the reviewer's questions is to be honest and explain the steps you will be taking to modify the patient's treatment. Do not try to mislead the reviewer or hide the facts of the case. When you are uncertain, openly acknowledge your uncertainty and state how you will gather more information so that you can effectively treat the patient. The most important thing is to demonstrate that you are aware of the patient's problems, are in control of the case, and have anticipated most eventualities. No ethical reviewer can expect you to do more than present a reasonable treatment plan and defend it.

When You and the Reviewer Disagree

At some point in the treatment of a patient, you and the reviewer are likely to disagree about whether the patient requires a specific level of care. In the last chapter, I described the appeal process that you can use if the reviewer does not approve care. Here I describe some of the specific clinical issues that commonly lead to disagreements about residential and inpatient care (Table 4–3). Subsequent chapters include discussion of the same issues as they apply to partial hospitalization and substance abuse rehabilitation. Disagreements between providers and reviewers generally revolve around one or more of the following issues: the severity of the patient's illness at the time of the review, estimates of the likelihood that the patient will benefit from the proposed treatment, the impact of the illness on the patient's ability to carry out the activities of daily life, and the type and intensity of clinical services the patient requires (see Case 4–3). As before, the provider's presentation of relevant clinical details often determines whether the reviewer approves or denies the requested care.

Case 4–3: Ben hit his brother

Clinical presentation: Ben is a 9-year-old boy who was hospitalized with a diagnosis of attention-deficit/hyperactivity disorder after he threatened his parents and hit his younger brother with a piece of wood. During a 4-day

Table 4-3.　Common areas of disagreement between provider and reviewer

- The severity of a patient's symptoms and their effect on his or her ability to function in daily life

- The potential effectiveness of additional treatment at the current level of care

- Whether the patient is likely to benefit from the current treatment

- Whether an unusual treatment is appropriate and effective

- Whether treatment with medication should be more aggressive

- Whether the patient is still suicidal or sufficiently psychotic to be a danger to himself or herself

- Whether the patient has an acute or chronic psychiatric disorder

hospitalization, Ben remained calm, attended classes, and complied with the hospital rules. The therapist asked for 4 more days. He argued that children take longer than adults to stabilize and that Ben was still too much of a danger to his family to return home without further treatment.

Reviewer's response: Ben appears to be stabilized and ready for discharge to an outpatient program. You must present specific information to substantiate your claim that Ben is still a danger to his family and requires additional hospitalization. Did he threaten to injure his brother again? Is he impulsive and angry? How do you explain Ben's calm, compliant behavior in the hospital? Does Ben have any insight into his aggressive behavior? How will you know when Ben is ready to be discharged? What objective measures will you use to make the determination? What type of treatment to prevent recurrence of the behavior has been arranged for Ben after discharge?

Many insurance and managed care companies stipulate that they provide benefits for the treatment of only acute illnesses, not chronic disorders that have little likelihood of improving with treatment. Therefore, a reviewer is likely to argue with you if you ask to admit a patient with dementia to a psychiatric unit. This does not necessarily mean that the reviewer will deny treatment. His or her approval often depends on how you define the clinical condition you are treating. Although Alzheimer's disease is a chronic illness, a patient with the illness may have acute exacerbations of delirium or psychosis superimposed on the dementia. Most insurance companies will cover treatment of the symptoms of delirium or psychosis but not the underlying memory loss caused by the dementia.

Given the distinction between acute and chronic disorders, it is advisable for you to highlight the patient's acute symptoms in your presentation to a reviewer. In other words, if one of your nursing home patients with Alzheimer's disease becomes so assaultive that he injures a staff member, you should emphasize control of the assaultive behavior, rather than the Alzheimer's disease, as the goal of inpatient treatment. This does not mean that you should ignore his memory problems inherent in the underlying disease. The patient's belligerence may be an expression of his anger and frustration with the disease and its effect on his life. Some supportive therapy might help him deal with the loss of his memories. In the early stages of the illness, supportive therapy may decrease or even eliminate the need for medication. Whether you decide to treat the patient with supportive therapy or medication, the most important thing to do, from the perspective of the reviewer, is to focus on the acute behavioral episode rather than the underlying chronic illness.

At some point in treatment, the acute symptoms of your patient with dementia will begin to diminish in intensity, and the reviewer will question the need for further inpatient care. You may think that the patient is not ready for discharge. If so, you need to provide specific examples of the patient's behavior during the prior 24 hours to support your argument. If, for example, the patient threw objects around his room or hit the staff, you could argue that he is still too agitated or assaultive to be managed at home or in a nursing facility. Few reviewers, however, will be convinced by a mere assertion, without relevant clinical examples, that the patient is not ready for discharge.

Even if a reviewer agrees that a patient has a psychiatric disorder that can benefit from treatment, he or she may disagree with the provider's decision about the level of care required. If the patient is in an inpatient unit, the reviewer may think he or she can be treated safely and effectively in a partial hospital program. If the patient is in a partial hospital program, the reviewer may think he or she can move to outpatient treatment. Your job is to provide the reviewer with the necessary clinical information to convince him or her that the patient requires the level of care you are requesting. To do this, you need to anticipate the reviewer's questions and respond to them in a reasonable fashion.

It is not uncommon for a practitioner to think he or she has provided sufficient information about a patient to support a request, only to have the reviewer deny further care. This usually occurs because the practitioner has not adequately described the patient's clinical condition. Frequently, a more detailed description of the patient's behavior and symptoms can convince a reviewer to change his or her mind and approve further care.

One practitioner requested additional hospital days for a young man experiencing a first psychotic episode. She explained that the patient appeared to be responding to internal stimuli and became suddenly aggressive without apparent provocation. "We're trying to stabilize his medication and help him develop some insight, some awareness of how sick he has been," she stated.

"Why can't you do that in a partial hospital program?" the reviewer asked.

"He's still too dangerous. If you could see him, you'd know what I mean," the clinician replied.

Because the clinician did not describe what she meant by *aggressive* or *dangerous* and the reviewer could not see the patient, he had little useful information on which to base his decision. The practitioner was essentially asking him to accept her judgment without being provided sufficient clinical data to determine whether the patient met the medical necessity criteria for continuing hospitalization. The reviewer later told me that he was about to deny further days of hospitalization but decided to ask the clinician to describe the patient in more detail.

"From what you have told me, this patient does not meet the medical necessity criteria for continued hospitalization," he told the clinician. "Can you describe him further?"

"He's so scary that the patients and staff are afraid to be alone in a room with him," she replied. "I've been in practice 15 years, and he is the scariest patient I've ever seen. His eyes dart around; he does not maintain eye contact. He's threatening. He's thrown furniture around the ward. He looks like he's going to explode at any minute."

"What's your treatment plan for the patient?" the reviewer asked.

"I want to give him enough medication to calm him and control his paranoid outbursts. Then we can transfer him to the partial hospital program."

The reviewer agreed with the plan and approved 3 additional days of hospitalization. The additional information that the clinician provided included more of the subtle details and conveyed more of the clinical flavor of the patient's condition than her initial description did. She succeeded in making the patient come alive for the reviewer. These observations helped the reviewer visualize the patient so that he could compare him with other paranoid and potentially dangerous patients he had seen in the past. Once that happened, he could understand and agree with her treatment plan. The clinician was lucky that the reviewer felt a responsibility to elicit more information. Other reviewers might have based their decision on the clinician's initial presentation of the patient's symptoms without asking for more details. Most reviewers think that it is the obligation of the clinician to forcefully defend his or her position.

Providing more details about a patient's clinical condition, however, will not always convince a reviewer to approve your request for care. The details you provide must be relevant to the level of care you are requesting. Suppose, for example, you are treating a man with schizophrenia whose main symptom is auditory hallucinations. The reviewer will want to know why the patient needs inpatient care, because many patients with schizophrenia have continuous auditory hallucinations but do not need hospitalization. The relevant details, in this case, would be the content and intensity of the hallucinations and the patient's response to them. If your patient hears voices that do not disturb him, do not significantly interfere with his ability to function, and do not command him to harm himself or another person, he will probably not meet the medical necessity criteria for hospitalization. Under these circumstances, it will not help to tell the reviewer the details of the voices—for instance, that they call the patient's name, mumble, or make irrelevant comments about his behavior. The reviewer will want to know why you cannot adjust the patient's medication in an outpatient setting.

Sometimes providers and reviewers disagree about the interpretation of the same symptom. In one case, a clinician called from a hospital emergency department to request admission for a patient who had stated that she was thinking of killing herself. The patient had been admitted for suicidal ideation to that facility and others many times before for a day or two. She had never made a serious suicide attempt. Nevertheless, the clinician considered the patient's suicidal ideation serious and believed she was a significant suicidal risk because she had stated that she would cut her wrists if she were discharged from the emergency department. The reviewer disagreed. He thought that the patient was manipulative and that there was no clear evidence that she was at risk of trying to kill herself. The practitioner and reviewer had opposite interpretations of the same clinical information. Under such circumstances, it may be useful to ask the reviewer what evidence he would need to decide that the patient met the medical necessity criteria for hospitalization. Even if his answer does not help resolve the current disagreement, it may help you understand how to present your next patient more successfully.

Suggested Reading

Bell CC, Clark DC: Violence among children and adolescents: adolescent suicide. Pediatr Clin North Am 45:356–380, 1998

Conwell Y: Management of suicidal behavior in the elderly. Psychiatr Clin North Am 20:667–683, 1997

Francis E, Marchand W, Hart M, et al: Utilization and outcome in an overnight psychiatric observation program at a Veterans Affairs medical center. Psychiatr Serv 51:92–95, 2000

Geller JL, Fisher WH, McDerneit M, et al: The effects of public managed care on patterns of intensive use of inpatient psychiatric services. Psychiatr Serv 51:1385–1391, 2000

Hughes DH: Suicide and violence assessment in psychiatry. Gen Hosp Psychiatry 18:416–421, 1996

Lansing AE, Lyons JS, Martens LC, et al: The treatment of dangerous patients in managed care: psychiatric hospital utilization and outcome. Gen Hosp Psychiatry 19:112–118, 1997

Moak GS: Geriatric psychiatry and managed care. Psychiatr Clin North Am 23:437–450, 2000

Neimeyer RA, Bonnelle K: The Suicide Intervention Response Inventory: a revision and validation. Death Stud 21:59–81, 1997

O'Donnell R, Rome D, Godin M, et al: Changes in inpatient psychiatric utilization and quality of care performance measures in a capitated HMO population, 1989–1999. Psychiatr Clin North Am 23:319–333, 2000

Orlando ML: Outcomes: essential information for clinical decision support: an interview with Ellen B. White. J Health Care Finance 24:71–81, 1998

Quinlivan RT: Treating high-cost users of behavioral health services in a health maintenance organization. Psychiatr Serv 51:159–161, 2000

Range LM, Knott EC: Twenty suicide assessment instruments: evaluation and recommendations. Death Stud 21:25–58, 1997

Rives W: Emergency department assessment of suicidal patients. Psychiatr Clin North Am 22:779–787, 1999

Rudd MD, Joiner TE: An integrative conceptual framework for assessing and treating suicidal behavior in adolescents. J Adolesc 21:489–498, 1998

Russ MJ, Kashdan T, Pollack S, et al: Assessment of suicide risk 24 hours after psychiatric hospital admission. Psychiatr Serv 50:1491–1493, 1999

Schnyder U, Valach L, Bichsel K, et al: Attempted suicide: do we understand the patients' reasons? Gen Hosp Psychiatry 21:62–69, 1999

Sulkowicz KJ: Psychodynamic issues in the emergency department. Psychiatr Clin North Am 22:911–922, 2000

CHAPTER 5

Presenting a Partial Hospital Case

Because the number of inpatient admissions and lengths of stay is rapidly decreasing to an irreducible minimum under the pressure of managed care, reviewers are beginning to focus more attention on lower levels of care, such as partial hospital and outpatient care, in which there still may be excess utilization and potential cost savings. Partial hospital programs, in particular, are under scrutiny. Although they provide less intense and therefore less expensive care for patients who do not need a full range of medical and multidisciplinary inpatient services, the cost of a partial hospital stay can rapidly increase as the days accumulate.

Many of the points raised in the discussion of inpatient presentations (Chapter 4) also apply to partial hospital cases. You must be willing to negotiate with the reviewer and to provide adequate clinical details to justify your requests for care. This is best done by answering four questions specific to partial hospital care (Table 5–1).

Why does the patient need partial hospital care now?   To answer the first question in Table 5–1, you must establish that your patient fulfills the medical necessity criteria for partial hospitalization (Table 5–2). The focus of partial hospital criteria, like that of the criteria for full, 24-hour hospitalization, is on the severity of the patient's illness and the intensity of the services required to treat the patient. To meet the criteria for partial hospitalization, the patient must have a DSM-IV-TR psychiatric disorder and there must be clear evidence that the patient either is a danger to self or others or is unable to care for himself or herself (see Case 5–1). In addition, you must demonstrate that the patient requires at least 4 hours of psychiatric and mul-

---

Table 5-1.   Four questions to answer in every partial hospital review

- Why does the patient need the structure and support of partial hospital treatment now?

- What is the goal of treatment and how will you know when you have accomplished it?

- How will you treat the patient?

- How will you maintain the patient's stability after discharge?

---

tidisciplinary care a day, 3–5 days a week. There is one major clinical difference between patients who require full hospitalization and those who require partial hospitalization. The former have little if any control over their symptoms and require 24-hour monitoring and treatment. The latter, on the other hand, either are able to control their symptoms by themselves when they are not in the treatment setting or have sufficient social and environmental support to help them do so.

Case 5–1: Kelly is promiscuous and irritable

Clinical presentation: Kelly is a 32-year-old woman with bipolar disorder who in the last 2 weeks has become sexually promiscuous and considerably more irritable and provocative than usual. Her outpatient therapist thinks that she probably stopped taking her medication. He is concerned that she will become frankly manic and require hospitalization unless she resumes taking the medication. The therapist wants to admit Kelly to a partial hospital program. Her family agrees to watch her in the evenings. The therapist's goal is to control Kelly's symptoms and help her gain some insight into the importance of continuing to take her medications. This goal will be achieved when Kelly becomes less irritable and sexually provocative and when her medication reaches a therapeutic blood level. The therapist estimates that this will take approximately 1 week in the partial hospital program.

Reviewer's response: Why can't Kelly restart her medication as an outpatient? Why can't the family monitor her medication? What evidence is there that Kelly is a danger to herself or unable to care for herself? Is she having unprotected sex with strangers? Has she provoked fights? Is she driving erratically? These would be evidence of her inability to care for herself. How will the partial hospital program staff help her gain insight into her illness? Does the hospital have special groups or programs that will help her gain insight?

Table 5-2.   Generic medical necessity criteria for partial hospitalization

- The patient must have a DSM-IV-TR psychiatric disorder that can be expected to benefit from inpatient treatment.

- There must be clear evidence that the patient is a danger to self or others or unable to care for himself or herself.

- The patient requires structured psychiatric and nursing care or supervision for approximately 4 hours a day.

- The patient has a supportive outside environment and is able to control the dangerous behavior when not in the hospital.

- The patient cannot be safely or effectively treated solely in an outpatient setting.

Because the criteria for partial hospitalization stipulate that a patient must control his or her symptoms outside the partial hospital setting, the first thing the reviewer will want to know is why your patient is unable to do so for the entire day. In other words, why cannot your patient be adequately treated and stabilized with more frequent outpatient visits? Many seasoned reviewers actually begin with a bias that most partial hospitalizations are unnecessary. They assume that if a patient requires only 3–5 days of partial hospital care a week, the patient is sufficiently intact to be treated in an intensive outpatient program at half the cost. Therefore, you must have a convincing reason why your patient requires the more intense, multidisciplinary services available in a partial hospital program and you must be able to explain how these services, and not outpatient treatment, specifically address the patient's symptoms. It is not sufficient to say that your patient is too unstable or sick to be treated solely on an outpatient basis.

Suppose, for example, you are treating a 23-year-old depressed woman with intermittent suicidal ideation and self-mutilating behavior in weekly outpatient therapy. The patient, whom I will call Nancy, made one suicide attempt by taking an overdose of 20 sleeping pills 6 months before and was hospitalized for 2 weeks. Until recently, weekly therapy sessions have helped her control the symptoms so that she can function at work and at home. Three weeks ago, her boyfriend of 1 year left her. Since that time, Nancy's suicidal ideation and intent have increased significantly. She calls you two or three times a week between sessions to tell you that she feels like killing herself and plans to take another overdose. She reports cutting herself on the thigh with a razor blade when she cannot reach you. When you provide extra therapy sessions and empathic support over the telephone, her symptoms diminish briefly, but they then reappear with the same intensity. You finally decide to admit her to a partial hospital program.

When you speak with the reviewer about this patient, you need to highlight those symptoms that not only are encompassed in the medical necessity criteria but can be expected to improve with the structure and support of a partial hospital program. Begin by giving a thumbnail description of the patient. Emphasize the escalation of Nancy's symptoms, including the active cutting behavior, the increased suicidal ideation, and the development of a suicide plan that is identical to one she acted on the year before. Give your assessment of the likelihood that the patient will act on her suicidal intent. Explain that you have tried to respond to these symptoms by providing additional therapy sessions but she continues to deteriorate. Describe other aspects of her behavior that exemplify the deterioration. Finally, tell the reviewer that you want to treat Nancy in a partial hospital program before her symptoms become so severe that you have to admit her to a 24-hour inpatient service. This last statement is especially important because most reviewers believe that the only reason for partial hospitalization is to provide sufficient structure and support to stabilize a patient's symptoms and avoid full hospitalization.

Because reviewers have become increasingly concerned about the inappropriate use of partial hospital services, common practices are coming under higher scrutiny. Some facilities, for example, routinely transfer inpatients to a partial hospital service before discharging them to outpatient care. Many of these patients, however, significantly improved during their stay on the inpatient service and do not meet the criteria for partial hospital care. Reviewers will generally approve partial hospital days if it appears that doing so will shorten the inpatient stay. They will not automatically approve the transition of every inpatient through a partial hospital program. Therefore, if you want to transfer your patient to a partial hospital program, you must have convincing evidence that the patient is still ill enough to meet the medical necessity criteria. It is not sufficient to argue that you want to slowly transition the patient to outpatient care.

In a similar sense, reviewers expect patients to meet the criteria for partial hospital care throughout their participation in the program. One provider initially received approval for 3 days of partial hospital care for his patient. The patient attended the first 2 days and then did not appear again for 10 days. At that time, the provider requested 3 additional days for the patient. The reviewer denied that request, reasoning that if the patient could maintain himself without partial hospital support for 10 days, he no longer needed that level of care. If you want the reviewer to approve further care, it is incumbent on you to provide sufficient clinical evidence to convince the reviewer that despite the patient's lack of compliance, he or she still requires partial hospital care.

Some reviewers are even more strict. They argue that if patients can function independently over the weekend without attending the program, they probably do not need further partial hospital care. This assumption may be correct if your patient is sufficiently intact that he or she spends her time working, relaxing, and socializing with other people over the weekend. Because few partial hospital patients function at that level, the best way to respond to the reviewer's challenge is to describe what your patient actually does when he or she is at home. One practitioner told the reviewer that his patient was so depressed that she had spent the entire weekend in bed, not getting up even to prepare meals or care for her children. Another practitioner reported that his irritable, hypomanic patient had to be continually supervised by a family member to ensure that he took his medication and did not get into arguments with neighbors and friends. Both practitioners' requests for additional days of care were approved because they effectively demonstrated that their patients were not ready to be transferred to outpatient care.

Reviewers generally expect physicians to reevaluate their patients whenever the patients are absent from the program for more than a couple of days, to determine whether they still need partial hospital care. This is part of the larger expectation that a physician be intimately involved in the patient's treatment. Reviewers reason that the major element that distinguishes partial hospital care from outpatient care is the need for intense, structured psychiatric, nursing, and multidisciplinary services. If the patient is sick enough to meet the criteria for a partial hospital program, he or she should be seen frequently, at least every other day, by the physician. Once this is no longer necessary, the patient should be discharged from the partial hospital program.

What is the goal of treatment? Once you have convinced the reviewer that the patient meets the medical necessity criteria for partial hospital care, you must answer the second question and explain what you are trying to accomplish with the partial hospital treatment. Several years ago, when I treated partial hospital patients, the program provided services that were very different from what they are today. At that time, the partial hospital program was filled with patients who had chronic psychiatric disorders. Many stayed in the program for weeks or months. One of the goals of the program was to socialize patients so that they could live alone or in groups outside the hospital. To do this, staff members often took patients to baseball games and movies or on shopping trips and bowling excursions. Socialization therapy, as we called it, may still exist somewhere, but it is not very common. Few contemporary insurance companies or reviewers would approve such an extended length of stay coupled with such a vague treatment plan.

Reviewers expect contemporary practitioners to be quite explicit about the clinical problems they are planning to treat and how they will treat them (see Case 5–2). To the reviewer, partial hospital programs are a means of providing intense care focused on specific clinical problems that are not serious enough to merit full hospitalization nor benign enough to be treated solely on an outpatient basis. When asked to authorize partial hospital care, the reviewer will try to determine whether the program provides the specific targeted care that the patient requires. In that sense, you should avoid using generic terms such as *coping* and *support* to describe what you are planning to do for the patient. These terms are so generic that they have no real therapeutic meaning. They suggest that you treat all patients the same.

Not supplying enough details was the mistake made by another clinician who had been treating a young man with anxiety and vague psychotic symptoms in a partial hospital program for 6 weeks. When the clinician requested 2 more weeks of care, the reviewer asked what he was trying to accomplish with the patient. The clinician stated, "He'll fall apart if I discharge him. He needs the support. He doesn't have anybody else." The reviewer asked him to be more specific. "The social worker has to hold his hand all day long," the clinician replied with some irritation. The reviewer refused to approve additional days of partial hospital care until the clinician specifically described what he was trying to accomplish in treatment other than "support" the patient. The clinician's initial plan was so vague that treatment could continue for weeks and months without a definitive conclusion being reached. The program was providing little more than what a friend or family member might do for the patient.

Case 5–2: Tony cut his mother

Clinical presentation: Tony is a 12-year-old depressed boy who in a fit of anger cut his mother with a knife. He was hospitalized for a week and discharged to an adolescent partial hospital program. The practitioner states that Tony is a potential danger to other students and cannot be sent directly back to school. The program will provide schooling for Tony so that he does not get behind in his studies.

Reviewer's response: What were the circumstances in which Tony cut his mother? Does he have a general problem controlling his impulses? Is he upset about what he did? Has he ever attacked a schoolmate? How will you determine that Tony is ready to be discharged from the partial hospital program? Is it sufficient for him to state that he will not hurt anyone again? How are you planning to explore and treat Tony's problems with his family? Is the family cooperating with Tony's treatment? When is the first family meeting? What other type of therapy are you providing for Tony? How will you evaluate the effect of the treatment? What type of follow-up care are you arranging for Tony when he is discharged?

It is important to remember that partial hospital care is not a long-term solution to any problem. If a patient's stay in a partial hospital program is extended beyond a reasonable period, it is usually an indication that important clinical problems have not been identified or resolved. This was evident in the case of Carol, a 45-year-old woman with metastatic cancer who was also struggling with issues of loss and separation. After a 3-day stay in an inpatient unit, Carol had been transferred to a partial hospital program, in which she was being treated for depression and suicidal ideation. She attended the program 5 days a week for 2 months. At the end of that time, her therapist requested an additional 2 months of partial hospital care, stating that the program was the only thing keeping the patient alive. He reported that the patient refused to undergo electroconvulsive therapy and was too "sensitive" to antidepressants to be treated with medication. Each time her therapist began to discuss discharge, the patient stated that she would kill herself if she had to leave the partial hospital program. The therapist was unable to describe what he was trying to accomplish other than prevent Carol from killing herself. He did not seem to recognize that her reluctance to leave the program was a significant problem that needed to be discussed in therapy and that was probably related to concerns about her illness as well as issues of separation from the partial hospital program. Rather than effectively treating her depression, the program and provider had fostered her dependency.

How should you describe your goals for a patient? Consider Nancy, the 23-year-old depressed patient discussed earlier. The reviewer will want to know exactly what you are planning to accomplish in the partial hospital program. Be explicit in your answer and refer to the patient's symptoms. Nancy's main problem is that she reacts to separations and disappointments with suicidal ideation and self-mutilating behavior. Tell the reviewer you are planning to target this problem by helping the patient learn other, more adaptive ways of dealing with separation. The goals of the partial hospitalization are to keep the patient safe until her suicidal and self-mutilating urges are diminished and to introduce her to therapy that can help her control these urges in the future. Explain that you can complete the first stage of this process only in the partial hospital program. That first stage will be accomplished when the patient is no longer feeling acutely suicidal and does not feel strong urges to cut herself.

Use the same tactics when you describe your treatment plan for other patients. If you are treating a schizophrenic man who has stopped taking his medications, tell the reviewer that you want to monitor his compliance with medication therapy while he attends support groups and classes that will help him understand the importance of such compliance. Explain that the patient will be ready for discharge when he begins to assume responsibility for taking his medication as prescribed. If your patient is a young woman with an eating disorder, argue that you want the staff to observe her eating two meals a day in the program while she participates in treatment groups focused on issues of self-esteem and body image. State that you will discharge the patient to outpatient care when she has gained a specific amount of weight and seems to be eating more normally.

How will you treat the patient?   Once you describe what you want to accomplish with treatment, you must specifically describe how you will treat the patient. In Nancy's case, you need to describe the specific modes of therapy you will use to address her suicidal ideation and self-mutilating behavior. You might, for example, decide to provide insight-oriented, cognitive, or group therapy to help her focus on the feelings associated with her loss and on her maladaptive response to those feelings. You might also wish to treat her fluctuating mood with a mood-stabilizing medication such as divalproex sodium. Whatever mode of therapy you choose, state your intentions and expectations for treatment as specifically and concisely as possible (see Case 5–3). You might, for example, present Nancy's treatment as follows:

> We will place the patient in a therapy group that meets five times a week and focuses on issues of low self-esteem, including the pain associated with blows to her self-esteem and methods she can use to protect herself from this pain. We will also provide individual cognitive-behavioral therapy that will focus on her extreme maladaptive and catastrophic response to separation and help her devise other, less destructive behaviors that she can use to manage these feelings. Finally, we will treat her with Depakote 250 mg three times a day and gradually increase the dose to the therapeutic blood level to determine whether this will stabilize her mood.

Case 5–3: Sandra's first psychotic episode

Clinical presentation: Sandra is an 18-year-old college student recently discharged from the hospital after a first psychotic episode that included auditory hallucinations, ideas of reference, and disorganized thinking. She responded moderately well to medication during her brief inpatient stay but still has some residual psychotic symptoms. Sandra can be managed at home when her parents are present. If left alone, however, she wanders out of the house and pesters people on the street with her bizarre philosophical theories. Sandra's psychiatrist admitted her to the partial hospital program to observe her, adjust her medications, and maintain her in a safe environment while her parents work. The psychiatrist's goal is to stabilize Sandra's residual symptoms with medications so that she can return to college or at least live more independently.

Reviewer's response: Do you expect to eradicate the patient's psychotic symptoms? How will you determine when the symptoms have stabilized? How long do you expect this to take? What medications will you prescribe and how will you adjust them? What will you do if your patient continues at her current level of functioning for a few weeks without change? What type of follow-up care are you arranging? How will you involve the family in your patient's treatment? What is the worst-case scenario for your patient and how would you handle it?

Reviewers are less likely to challenge you if you are confident in your presentation, appear to be in command of the patient's clinical details, and are certain about the validity of your therapy and your patient is responding to treatment. The last condition is the most important. Every reviewer eventually expects to see evidence that your patient is benefiting from treatment. If your patient is not responding, the reviewer will want to know why and what you are planning to do about it. Whatever you say, do not tell the reviewer that there is nothing more you can do except continue the current treatment. No reviewer will accept that answer.

That was exactly the problem with Carol's treatment. Let us assume that she was your patient and you argued that because she became suicidal whenever the issue of discharge was raised, you had no option other than to keep her in the partial hospital program. To the reviewer, it would seem as though you did not know how to treat the patient, because you appeared to be unaware of the critical clinical issues related to her depression and periodic suicidal ideation. You could allay the reviewer's concerns by presenting a brief analysis of the patient's main clinical problems and an aggressive treatment plan detailing how you will address these problems:

This patient is a 45-year-old depressed woman who has advanced, possibly terminal, cancer. She is very dependent on the partial hospital program and strongly resists discharge. I plan to help her explore her feelings about her illness, her fears of impending death, and her difficulty in leaving the program. Tomorrow, I will begin intensive individual psychotherapy focusing on her illness and concerns about death. I will also enroll her in a hospital-sponsored support group for patients with advanced cancer. Finally, I have discussed the patient's case with her psychiatrist and he has decided to start low-dose sertraline therapy and slowly increase the dose. If she develops side effects, he will try other antidepressant medications until he finds one she can tolerate. We are requesting six additional sessions of partial hospital care to implement this treatment plan.

The average reviewer would probably approve three or four sessions, rather than the six you requested. At the end of that time, he or she would expect you to report on the patient's clinical progress and indicate when you thought the patient would be discharged.

To a great extent, the decision about when to discharge a patient depends on your expectations for partial hospital treatment in general and your specific therapeutic goals for the patient. Because this is one of the main areas of conflict between providers and reviewers, it is important for you to understand the reviewer's theoretical attitude toward partial hospital care as a method of treatment. Most reviewers believe that partial hospitalization is a temporary therapeutic solution that may help patients focus on specific clinical problems until those problems have improved sufficiently to be treated at a less intense level of care. The emphasis is on improvement, not resolution. The expectation that every patient's problems will be completely resolved before discharge from a partial hospital program is unrealistic.

Given this point of view, the reviewer may decide that your patient is ready for discharge from the partial hospital program before you do. If you disagree, you will have to present a reasonable argument—one that is based on the patient's symptoms and the medical necessity criteria—that your patient needs additional days of care. The most convincing argument you can make is that if your patient is discharged too soon, he or she may have a relapse and require readmission to the program. This is an especially effective argument if you have evidence that the patient relapsed in the past under similar circumstances. If you do not have such evidence, you will have to demonstrate the patient's continuing instability by citing examples of his or her current symptoms. Although reviewers want to have patients discharged as fast as possible, they are also aware that it is more expensive to readmit a patient than to continue partial hospital care for a few additional days.

How will you maintain the patient's stability after discharge? Be aware that providers and reviewers tend to have different views about the cause of relapses. Providers commonly believe that their partial hospital patients relapse because they are discharged prematurely. Reviewers, on the other hand, believe that patients relapse mainly because they do not have effective follow-up care. At the same time, reviewers believe that providers often cite the difficulty of arranging follow-up care as an excuse for trying to prolong a patient's stay in a partial hospital program. This seeming contradiction is resolved when it is remembered that one of the reviewer's concerns is to decrease the use of clinical care by increasing its efficiency. One way to improve efficiency is to make sure that appropriate follow-up care is available when the patient is ready for discharge. This means that ideally you should begin working on discharge plans as soon as your patient is admitted. This is particularly important for patients with chronic psychiatric disorders who have frequent exacerbations of their symptoms.

Why worry about a few patients with chronic disorders and frequent exacerbations? The reason is simple. These patients use an enormous amount of health care resources relative to their proportion of the population. A small number are readmitted to various facilities 5, 10, or 20 times a year. Reviewers understand, better than the average practitioner does, that effectively treating and stabilizing these patients in an outpatient setting will substantially reduce the overall use of expensive full and partial hospital services. Surprisingly, the bulk of these patients share a few common problems. Many are lonely, depressed, and hopeless, with fluctuating self-esteem and periodic suicidal ideation and self-destructive behavior. They view the partial hospital program as an oasis in the midst of lives of loneliness and despair. Others have mood instability and oscillate among mania, hypomania, and depression. Still others have significant problems with interpersonal relationships or have fluctuating psychotic symptoms. These are the patients that concern reviewers the most, because they are at high risk for readmission.

Unfortunately, the transition of care for such patients is not always well planned, as the discharge instructions for one such patient demonstrated. They stated: "Call the hospital or your physician when you have suicidal thoughts or feel that you will hurt yourself again." There was no evidence in the patient's record that any comprehensive therapeutic plan had been developed to treat her and provide the broad-based support she would probably need after her discharge. When her symptoms flared up again, her psychiatrist would probably have no recourse other than to readmit her to the partial hospital program.

Curiously, even good clinicians forget about the importance of effective continuity of care. I raised the issue once while reviewing the records of a partial hospital program in an excellent hospital. The staff of the program had readmitted a patient with suicidal ideation four times in 3 months. When I asked the medical director what programs they had developed to maintain the patient's stability after discharge, he seemed surprised. As far as he was concerned, his responsibility ended once the patient was discharged. He apparently thought of mental health care as a series of discrete responses to disconnected episodes of illness rather than a continuum of services that provided what the patient needed at different stages of his or her illness. Without sufficient outpatient support, the patient's readmission was predictable. Many health care systems are organized to provide intense care during a crisis and less adequate care during the intervening periods between crises. The problem occurs in even the best hospitals, because the staff take it for granted that these patients will need frequent readmissions.

Ignoring continuity of care with such patients can sometimes have dramatic, if not embarrassing, consequences. I learned that lesson several years ago when I was the medical director of a partial hospital program that occupied one wing of a locked psychiatric unit. One day I admitted an anxious, depressed, angry, and moderately paranoid young woman. I started low-dose antipsychotic therapy and her paranoia quickly resolved. During the remainder of her stay, she was demanding, refused treatment, criticized her care, antagonized and manipulated other patients, and developed a hostile-dependent relationship with me and the staff. Despite her protests, I finally discharged her 2 weeks later and referred her to a nearby community mental health center for follow-up outpatient treatment. I made no attempt to have her establish some sort of relationship, however tenuous, with the staff of the mental health center before her discharge. That was my undoing. The morning after her discharge, I was sitting in the nursing station and heard a commotion. I turned and saw my former patient standing outside the ward, pounding on the locked glass door and screaming to be let in. Her transition to outpatient care had apparently not gone smoothly.

What did I do wrong? Among other things, I had responded to my patient's hostility and neglected to address her dependency needs. I had offered her a referral to a generic mental health clinic without connecting her to an individual who might help her in her continuing struggle with intense loneliness and despair. I was just like the medical director of the partial hospital program who thought his responsibility to the patient ended the moment she was referred and walked out his door. There was more than a little moral tinge to my attitude toward the patient, a sense that it was about time she handled some of her problems by herself. On some level, I am sure she detected my attitude, and she publicly exacted her revenge.

It is one thing to say that every such patient with frequent exacerbations should have effective follow-up care. It is an entirely different thing to identify and arrange the appropriate type of care. In the case of Nancy, the 23-year-old woman with depression and suicidal ideation, the goal of partial hospitalization is to treat the acute symptoms until they have ameliorated sufficiently for her to be safely discharged to outpatient care. Long before that happens, a good reviewer will ask you about your plans for the patient's follow-up care. He or she will want to know what type of care Nancy will receive and how the transition from partial hospital care to that care will be managed. A routine referral to an outpatient clinic will not satisfy the reviewer. Think about what your patient needs. You know that once she leaves the partial hospital program, with its multiple activities, structured days, and attentive staff, she will feel empty and abandoned. There must be something to replace that support, or her sense of emptiness and abandonment may become so strong that she again feels suicidal. Weekly therapy and periodic visits to her outpatient psychiatrist for medication checks will not be sufficient to help her master her feelings.

What should you tell the reviewer? Describe your discharge plans for your patient during the initial discussion with the reviewer:

> The patient is a 23-year-old woman who was admitted to our partial hospital program for the second time in 6 months with suicidal ideation and self-mutilating behavior precipitated by a breakup with her boyfriend. After we discharge her, this patient will need a great deal of support to help her master her chronic problems of poor self-esteem, separation anxiety, and self-destructive behavior. We plan to refer her for cognitive-behavioral therapy to help her learn how to control her periodic urges to hurt herself before they reach crisis proportions. Her outpatient psychiatrist will manage her medications. In addition, we propose to enroll her in a special crisis group that will provide her with more intense outpatient support when her symptoms flare up. Our goal is to provide enough outpatient support to help the patient weather her crises without hospitalization until she learns how to manage her urges on her own.

Reviewers are impressed with clinicians who can succinctly describe their patients' clinical problems and present logical treatment plans that take into account the patients' immediate and long-term therapeutic needs. The secret of a successful partial hospital review is to seize the initiative in your discussion with the reviewer and anticipate his or her questions. Once you have established your credibility with the reviewer, he or she will probably review fewer of your cases, and those in a more perfunctory manner.

Suggested Reading

Creed F, Mbaya P, Lancashire S, et al: Cost effectiveness of day and inpatient psychiatric treatment: results of a randomised controlled trial. BMJ 314:1381–1385, 1997

Simpson EB, Pistorello J, Begin A, et al: Focus on women: use of dialectical behavior therapy in a partial hospital program for women with borderline personality disorder. Psychiatr Serv 49:669–673, 1998

Sledge WH, Tebes J, Rakfeldt J, et al: Day hospital/crisis respite care versus inpatient care, part I: clinical outcomes. Am J Psychiatry 153:1065–1073, 1996

Sledge WH, Tebes J, Wolff N, et al: Day hospital/crisis respite care versus inpatient care, part II: service utilization and costs. Am J Psychiatry 153:1074–1083, 1996

CHAPTER 6

Presenting a Substance Abuse Case

Insurance companies and reviewers tend to be skeptical, or perhaps ambivalent, about substance-related disorders, because their treatment is so different from that required for other types of mental illness. Substance abuse treatment has traditionally been divided into two distinct but overlapping stages, detoxification and rehabilitation. The goal of detoxification is to wean the patient from the substance or substances the patient is dependent on, without provoking a painful or dangerous withdrawal. The goal of rehabilitation is to decrease the individual's craving for an abused substance and help him or her establish and maintain abstinence from that substance. Disputes usually arise over whether an individual needs formal substance abuse treatment and, if so, the type and intensity of service the patient requires. The best way to convince a reviewer that your patient needs substance abuse treatment is to answer the same four questions discussed in earlier chapters (Table 6–1). These questions apply equally well to inpatient detoxification and to residential substance abuse rehabilitation.

Substance Abuse Detoxification

Why does the patient need inpatient detoxification now?   Because it is a medically monitored process, detoxification generally provokes fewer disagreements between providers and reviewers than does rehabilitation. The physical signs and symptoms of alcohol and opiate withdrawal are straightforward, reasonably consistent, and readily acknowledged by most clinicians. A patient's detoxification is individualized and dictated by his or her

---

Table 6-1.   Four questions to answer in every substance abuse review

- Why does the patient need inpatient detoxification or residential substance abuse rehabilitation now?

- What is the goal of treatment and how will you know when you have accomplished it?

- How will you treat the patient?

- How will you maintain the patient's abstinence after discharge?

---

signs and symptoms. Disputes usually center around the necessity, timing, and duration of inpatient detoxification. Addiction specialists believe that detoxification, especially for heavy alcohol and drug abusers, can be undergone more safely and effectively in the hospital. Reviewers are reluctant to approve inpatient detoxification, because it is expensive and because they believe that few patients require 24-hour hospital care to manage their withdrawal. They argue that a substantial amount of alcohol and drug detoxification occurs on the streets without medical intervention, or with minimal medical supervision in outpatient, partial hospital, or residential programs. There are, however, certain types of withdrawal that require hospitalization. These are defined in the medical necessity criteria for inpatient detoxification (Table 6–2). If you want to detoxify a substance-dependent patient in the hospital, you must answer the first question in Table 6–1 by demonstrating that your patient meets these medical necessity criteria (see Case 6–1).

Case 6–1: "I want to stop drinking now!"

Clinical presentation: Curtis is a 27-year-old single man who drinks a pint of liquor a day. His girlfriend has told him that she will leave him if he does not stop drinking now. Curtis spoke with his employee assistance program representative, who referred him to a local hospital emergency department for admission to the detoxification unit. The substance abuse counselor at the detoxification program called for approval to admit Curtis.

Reviewer's response: Has Curtis tried to stop drinking before on his own? If so, what happened? If he hasn't tried to stop, why can't he gradually cut back on his drinking by himself? Has Curtis tried outpatient detoxification? Has he spoken with his primary care physician about stopping? Is there anything that might complicate Curtis's withdrawal? Does he have a

---

Table 6-2. Generic medical necessity criteria for inpatient alcohol or drug detoxification

---

- The patient has used alcohol or drugs heavily for an extended period.

- There is the potential for serious physical harm to the patient due to withdrawal from the abused substance.

- The patient has signs and symptoms of withdrawal.

- The patient cannot be safely detoxified on an outpatient basis.

- The patient requires 24-hour medical treatment to manage his or her withdrawal.

---

history of seizures or blackouts? Does he have a debilitating illness that would make withdrawal particularly dangerous? Does he have signs or symptoms of withdrawal? If there are no complicating factors, he doesn't meet medical necessity criteria for inpatient detoxification. We would approve him for outpatient detoxification.

Most medical necessity criteria for detoxification stipulate that individuals be hospitalized only if they are at risk for significant physical harm or death from withdrawal without immediate medical treatment. The criteria usually include three general circumstances in which withdrawal may be dangerous enough for the patient to require hospitalization. The first is when there is reasonable evidence to suggest that the patient's withdrawal will be severe. If, for example, an individual has been drinking heavily and presents for treatment with a significantly increased blood pressure and temperature, there is a high likelihood that he or she is in the early stages of delirium tremens, a potentially fatal illness. The second circumstance is when the patient has a medical illness that will complicate withdrawal. In one case, a 65-year-old woman who had been drinking a fifth of whiskey a day was found to have a lymphoma. She was admitted for inpatient detoxification when her oncologist explained that he could not start chemotherapy until she was completely withdrawn from alcohol. The third circumstance is when a patient experienced complications, such as delirium tremens or seizures, during a prior detoxification.

Two equally qualified practitioners may differ in their interpretation of medical necessity criteria for the same patient. This is particularly true of cases in which it is difficult to be certain that the patient is at risk for serious physical harm. Suppose that you request inpatient alcohol detoxification for a man with a blood pressure of 150/90 mm Hg and mild tremors, your reason being that the individual is in imminent delirium tremens. The reviewer may respond that the patient does not need to be hospitalized because his blood pressure is only slightly above normal and many alcohol-abusing patients experience tremors without progressing into delirium tremens. You and the reviewer are obviously interpreting the same data differently based on your clinical experience and roles. You believe that your patient should be hospitalized even if there is only a small chance that he will have a dangerous detoxification. The reviewer, on the other hand, believes that the patient should not be hospitalized, because there is only a small chance that he will have a dangerous detoxification. The important question is, how can the dispute be resolved? You might suggest that your patient be admitted to a 23-hour bed for observation and treatment. If the patient shows further symptoms of severe withdrawal during that time, he will be admitted to the hospital. If not, he will be managed as an outpatient. A reasonable reviewer will agree with this treatment plan.

Reviewers are obligated to approve inpatient detoxification for patients who meet the medical necessity criteria. If, however, the patient has had multiple detoxifications and relapses in the recent past, the reviewer may argue that the patient should not undergo another inpatient detoxification, because he or she will probably begin drinking again. If the reviewer does present this argument, tell him or her that it is your understanding that the decision to hospitalize is based solely on the medical necessity criteria and that those criteria do not exclude patients who have relapsed several times in the past. The problem of multiple detoxifications is an issue of insurance benefits, not clinical decisions. If a patient has medical benefits that cover an unlimited number of detoxifications, the patient is entitled to them as long as he or she meets the medical necessity criteria. The way to reduce the number of future detoxifications is to make sure that the patient receives the necessary follow-up care to maintain abstinence.

It is far easier to convince a reviewer that a patient requires inpatient detoxification for alcohol than it is to obtain approval of inpatient detoxification for opiates or other drugs. Opiate withdrawal, although uncomfortable, is rarely dangerous unless there are complicating factors. Given reviewer bias, you need to present convincing clinical data that will justify your request to hospitalize a patient for opiate detoxification. It is not sufficient to argue that your patient is addicted to large amounts of heroin or Vicodin (hydrocodone bitartrate and acetaminophen). The reviewer will argue that withdrawal from even heavy doses of such drugs can be safely accomplished on an outpatient basis. Instead, focus on those elements of the patient's condition that might place him or her in significant physical jeopardy. If, for example, your patient has uncontrollable diarrhea, you might argue that he or she will develop a severe electrolyte imbalance without 24-hour medical monitoring and intravenous fluids. Be prepared, however, to provide the reviewer with your patient's latest electrolyte values and to describe what you have done to control the diarrhea.

You might also be able to argue that your patient meets the medical necessity criteria for inpatient detoxification because he or she is abusing large amounts of several classes of substances at the same time. In the following case, the provider was able to demonstrate that the patient's addiction was so complex that she could be safely detoxified only in the hospital.

> Sally is a 31-year-old single woman with persistent headaches and chronic back pain that began after she was involved in a car accident 3 years earlier. She has had several comprehensive medical evaluations, but physicians have not been able to discover any physical basis for her pain. Sally has been unable to work and has become increasingly anxious and depressed since the accident. She is being treated by her primary care physician, who prescribes medication for her pain, anxiety, and depression. Sally also makes at least one emergency department visit a month, during which she receives additional prescriptions for Demerol and Ativan. Her primary care physician has tried to help her detoxify from her pain medications several times, but without success. Sally became scared that her drug use was out of control when she experienced a brief blackout while waiting in her car at a stoplight. She awoke to find a line of cars and trucks honking at her. After that episode, Sally came to our hospital and asked for help to decrease the amount of drugs she is taking. She estimates that she is taking Dilaudid 80 mg, Xanax 4 mg, Effexor 75 mg, and varying amounts of Ativan, Fiorinal, and Demerol each day.

The reviewer approved inpatient detoxification for Karen because she had failed multiple attempts at supervised outpatient detoxification and was at risk for seizures from benzodiazepine withdrawal as well as severe symptoms from opiate withdrawal.

What is the goal of treatment? How will you treat the patient? The second and third questions in Table 6–1 can be answered together. The goal of detoxification is to withdraw an individual from addicting substances without provoking severe, potentially life-threatening side effects. That goal is accomplished when the individual is no longer using drugs or alcohol and is no longer experiencing significant symptoms of withdrawal. Clinicians, however, frequently disagree about the end point of treatment and how long the patient needs to stay in the hospital. That decision depends on the patient's symptoms. Typically, reviewers question the last day of hospitalization for a patient undergoing alcohol detoxification. Addiction specialists commonly want to see their patients completely free of symptoms before discharge. Reviewers, on the other hand, emphasize that the potential for serious physical harm is the main criterion for continued hospitalization. They believe that a patient can be discharged once his or her major physiological indices are normal, even if the patient still feels mildly ill. The residual mild symptoms, they argue, can be treated in a rehabilitation program. The question, of course, is what constitutes a mild symptom. If your patient's vital signs are normal but he or she is still tremulous, nauseated, vomiting, or having multiple episodes of diarrhea during the day, you might argue that the patient is still too sick to be able to benefit from a rehabilitation program.

How will you maintain the patient's abstinence after discharge?   Once your patient is adequately detoxified, you need to address the fourth question and explain how you will help the patient maintain his or her abstinence after discharge from your program. Providers typically respond that they will transfer the patient to a rehabilitation program. This makes sense because there is little time during detoxification to work with the patient on issues of abstinence. Reviewers will generally accept this answer unless the patient has undergone multiple prior trials of rehabilitation.

Substance Abuse Rehabilitation

It is more difficult to explain why a patient needs substance abuse rehabilitation than why an individual requires detoxification, because the indications for rehabilitation are more subjective and harder to verify than those for detoxification. I focus on residential rehabilitation in this chapter because reviewers and providers tend to disagree more about an individual's need for residential treatment than about the need for any other type of rehabilitation.

Why does the patient need residential rehabilitation now?   As with detoxification, you can best answer the first question in Table 6–1 by demonstrating that the patient meets the medical necessity criteria for that treatment (Table 6–3).

Most medical necessity criteria for residential rehabilitation stipulate that the patient have a history of recent, active, heavy substance use that

Table 6-3.   Generic medical necessity criteria for residential alcohol or
drug rehabilitation

- The patient has an active history of substance use that
  meets DSM-IV-TR diagnostic criteria for substance
  abuse or dependence.

- The individual is unable to maintain abstinence.

- The individual has failed outpatient treatment or there
  are circumstances that would make it difficult or impossible for outpatient treatment to be effective.

- The individual is mentally capable of participating in
  the rehabilitation program and will do so voluntarily.

- There is evidence that the individual will benefit from
  treatment and remain abstinent.

meets DSM-IV-TR criteria for substance abuse or dependence. It is not sufficient, however, simply to tell the reviewer that your patient's substance use
meets DSM-IV-TR criteria. You need to provide the reviewer with answers to
the same questions a colleague might ask if you were to refer the patient to
him or her. How heavy is the patient's substance use? Does he or she drink
five beers a day, or a fifth of vodka? Does the patient use the substance every
day or only occasionally? How long has he or she been using drugs or alcohol? Has the patient ever experienced blackouts or delirium tremens? Has
the drug or alcohol use produced any serious medical problems? Does the
patient have any legal problems associated with the substance abuse? Has
the patient lost his or her job or is the patient having problems at work because of the substance abuse? When did he or she last use drugs or alcohol?
Does the patient truly understand that he or she has to stop using drugs or
alcohol? Why does the patient want to stop now? Has something recently
changed in the patient's life that makes him or her want to stop? The answers
to these questions provide important information about the depth of your
patient's addiction, its effect on his or her life, and your patient's ability to
control the addiction. They add additional weight to the DSM-IV-TR diagnosis and help convince the reviewer that your patient needs residential rehabilitation.

The main indication for substance abuse rehabilitation is an individual's inability to remain abstinent. Yet this is often one of the most difficult things to establish. It is not sufficient for an individual simply to state that he or she has difficulty remaining abstinent, just as it is not sufficient for a patient to state that he or she feels suicidal. You must elicit more detailed clinical information to substantiate the patient's claim (see Case 6–2). If the patient is addicted to alcohol, has he or she ever tried to stop drinking on his or her own? What happened when the individual tried to stop? Is it more difficult for him or her to remain abstinent in some life situations than in others? Does the patient drink when alone at home or when surrounded by other people? Does he or she spend time with people who do not drink? Can the individual control his or her drinking at those times? Does he or she compensate by drinking more later? Does the patient wake up in the morning with the shakes and need a drink to get started? Is there any particular time of day that he or she is more likely to drink, or is it spread throughout the day? The reviewer is looking for evidence that the individual's drug or alcohol use is so persistent and out of control that he or she needs treatment to abstain.

Case 6–2: Mary stopped drinking on her own

Clinical presentation: Mary is a 37-year-old woman who has been abusing alcohol for 10 years. She drank approximately six to eight beers a day until a month ago, when she made a promise to her dying mother that she would stop drinking. Mary has never had any substance abuse rehabilitation treatment. She recently saw her internist for a physical examination and mentioned that she was afraid that she was going to start drinking again. The internist requested approval to admit her to a residential rehabilitation program to help her stay sober.

Reviewer's response: Why does this patient need residential rehabilitation? She is obviously motivated to remain abstinent, because she has done so for a month on her own. She will always have an urge to drink. Is there any evidence that she is going to begin drinking again now? Has something recently changed in her life that would make her more likely to begin drinking? Is she attending Alcoholics Anonymous? Given her motivation, this patient will probably be able to maintain her abstinence with outpatient therapy. She currently does not meet the criteria for residential alcohol rehabilitation. Such an admission could actually undermine her own considerable efforts to remain abstinent.

The determination of an individual's inability to remain abstinent is also complicated by the difference between substance abuse symptoms and symptoms of other psychiatric disorders. Patients do not consciously choose to become anxious, depressed, or psychotic. Substance abusers, however, make a voluntary choice to use an addicting substance. Clinicians maintain that addicted patients have no control over that choice because of their intense craving for the abused substance. Reviewers, however, argue that craving is a very subjective symptom that is difficult to verify. They tend to be skeptical of the claim that an individual patient is unable to control his or her use of an addicting substance, unless there is a preponderance of evidence supporting that conclusion. You need to provide such convincing information to the reviewer. Arguments about a patient's ability to remain abstinent are a common area of disagreement between providers and reviewers (Table 6–4).

Disagreements during evaluation commonly stem from different clinical interpretations of the inability to maintain abstinence. These differences are evident in the case of Hal, a 38-year-old married man who had been installing carpets for a local flooring company for 6 years. When he started working, Hal could carpet an average-size living room in less than an hour. That was before he began drinking heavily. Initially, Hal drank a beer or two with friends after work. Gradually his drinking increased. He had a beer for lunch, then two or three. Within a few months, he was drinking several cans of beer a day. Soon Hal's customers called to complain. The seams between sections of carpet he installed were crooked with noticeable gaps. Here and there, tufts protruded from the molding. The company's personnel director warned Hal that he would be fired if he drank on the job. Hal managed to stop drinking on his own for 2 weeks. At the end of that time, he saw his primary care physician, who called for approval to admit Hal to a residential rehabilitation program.

"Why does he need residential rehabilitation?" the reviewer asked.

"He can't stop drinking," the physician replied.

"He's been abstinent for 2 weeks. That's good evidence that he can control his drinking if he wants to. He may be a good candidate for outpatient rehabilitation."

"He says that he's having trouble not drinking."

"It's a day-to-day thing. He needs to work on it 1 day at a time. What evidence do you have that he can't continue his abstinence?"

"Just what he tells me."

"I'm sorry, I can't approve residential rehabilitation for your patient just because he's afraid he may start drinking again."

Many substance abuse clinicians would disagree with the reviewer's decision. They would argue that Hal was obviously motivated to stop drinking and was struggling to maintain his abstinence. They would complain that

Table 6-4.   Potential areas of disagreement about substance abuse
rehabilitation

- **Patient's ability to abstain:** Can the patient abstain on
  his or her own some part of the day, or does the patient
  require 24-hour support from a residential program?

- **Patient's motivation:** Is the patient truly convinced that
  he or she has a serious substance abuse problem and
  needs rehabilitation? If not, how will the patient's denial
  be addressed?

- **Patient's potential for relapse:** Has the patient had prior
  relapses? Does he or she have a high likelihood of relapsing again? What is the program doing to respond to
  the potential for relapse?

- **Patient's ability to participate in the program:** Can the
  patient participate actively in the rehabilitation program? Is he or she cognitively impaired or too ill to participate?

- **Level of care needed:** Does the patient need residential
  rehabilitation, or can he or she be treated in an outpatient
  program?

- **Provision of individualized treatment:** Does the rehabilitation program provide the same treatment for every
  patient, or does it individualize in response to each patient's needs?

- **End point of residential rehabilitation treatment:** Does
  the program have specific criteria for deciding when a
  patient is ready for discharge, or do the program staff try
  to keep the patient as long as possible?

- **Type of treatment:** Does the program provide an acceptable amount of individual, group, and family therapy led
  by highly trained and credentialed therapists?

- **Appropriateness of treatment:** Does the program rely
  on atypical treatments such as equine therapy, rock
  climbing therapy, or wilderness experience therapy?

rather than responding to Hal's success with additional support, the reviewer used that success as evidence to deny more intense treatment. The reviewer, however, may have simply reasoned that if Hal could remain abstinent on his own for 2 weeks, he could continue to do so with the help of outpatient treatment.

Are there any extenuating factors that might convince a reviewer to approve residential rehabilitation under these circumstances? Suppose Hal's wife had announced, 2 days before Hal saw his primary care provider, that she was leaving him. You could argue that the stress of separation and the lack of support from his wife would make it difficult for Hal to maintain his abstinence without more intense treatment. Any such recent, dramatic change in Hal's life might convince the reviewer to approve residential rehabilitation, if you provided adequate evidence suggesting that the event would decrease Hal's ability to remain abstinent.

Suppose that instead of having a long history of steady drinking followed by a brief period of sobriety, your patient drank in binges. That was the situation for Bill, an 18-year-old college student who went on weekend drinking sprees a couple of times a month. In between, he remained sober. Early one morning, after a binge, he arrived in the emergency department with a deep cut in his thigh. Bill could not remember how he had been injured, but a friend reported that he had fallen on a beer bottle during a party in his fraternity house. The physician who attended to Bill's wound requested approval to admit him to a residential rehabilitation program. The reviewer responded that Bill was able to abstain on his own between binges and could be treated with outpatient counseling and Alcoholics Anonymous meetings. The physician disagreed. How could he convince the reviewer to change his mind? He could argue that Bill was a young student with no history of treatment and it was worth providing him with more intense rehabilitation now to prevent a lifetime of alcohol abuse. He might also argue that there was a great deal of drinking in the fraternity house where Bill lived and it would be difficult for him to stay abstinent if he remained there. A reasonable reviewer might agree to this request if the physician could demonstrate that the rehabilitation program would address Bill's specific problem of binge drinking, that it would not be easy to find him another place to live where he would not be continually exposed to drinking, and that the admission to a residential rehabilitation program would not seriously disrupt his life by forcing him to drop out of school.

Providers and reviewers frequently disagree about whether a patient needs residential or outpatient rehabilitation (see Case 6–3). Substance abuse clinicians generally believe that every individual has a far better chance of becoming and staying abstinent if he or she is treated in a residential program. Many medical necessity criteria, however, stipulate that an individual first undergo a trial of outpatient rehabilitation, unless there is a high likelihood that outpatient rehabilitation will fail. If you believe that your patient needs residential rehabilitation, you will have to convince the reviewer that the patient is likely to fail in an outpatient program. The two most effective arguments are that the individual lives in an environment that is not conducive to abstinence and that he or she is a danger to self or others because of the substance abuse. If the individual lives with other substance abusers, you could argue that it would be very difficult for him or her to remain abstinent at home. You could also argue that the individual is a danger to other people when he or she drinks or uses drugs because the individual becomes violent or insists on driving. In either case, be prepared to provide evidence from family, friends, or other sources that supports your argument.

Case 6–3: "Why does he need residential treatment?"

Clinical presentation: Tom is a 47-year-old employed, married man with a supportive family. He has a history of alcohol abuse. He has been sober for the last 9 months, since he underwent a course of outpatient alcohol rehabilitation. Three days ago, he began drinking again. His Alcoholics Anonymous sponsor wants him admitted to a 24-hour substance abuse rehabilitation program for treatment.

Reviewer's response: Why did the patient start drinking again? What changed in his life? Why does he need inpatient alcohol rehabilitation? He did well for 9 months after outpatient rehabilitation. Is he motivated to quit again? Given that he lives in a supportive family environment where there is no alcohol abuse, why can't the patient be treated again in an outpatient program?

To benefit from rehabilitation, a patient must be mentally capable of participating in the program. If your patient has some cognitive impairment, you need to convince the reviewer that he or she will still be able to benefit from educational sessions and group therapy. One way to demonstrate this is to present specific information from your mental status examination of the patient that demonstrates his or her capacity to learn new information and think critically. If there is continuing concern about the patient's cognitive capacity, you can order psychological testing.

An individual must eventually accept that he or she needs treatment for substance abuse if he or she is to derive benefit from a rehabilitation program (see Case 6–4). This is a particular problem for individuals who are ordered into treatment by the courts. The ultimate goal of rehabilitation is to help individuals voluntarily abstain from using substances. Reviewers ask, "How can an individual be expected to abstain from alcohol or drugs in the future if that individual is not voluntarily participating in his or her own rehabilitation?" Many substance abuse clinicians would argue that this is not a valid question. They maintain that an individual's unwillingness to freely participate in a program is probably a sign of denial and that breaking down denial is one of the major goals of treatment. Reviewers respond that a patient's denial must be sufficiently overcome before he or she enters rehabilitation if the process is to have any hope of success. They add that if an individual is still denying the need for treatment, he or she is not ready for it.

Case 6–4: Jerry needs more intense care

Clinical presentation: Jerry is a 15-year-old boy who abuses alcohol and marijuana. His father brought him to the hospital to be evaluated for treatment. The addictionologist recommended that Jerry be admitted to a partial hospital substance abuse rehabilitation program. Jerry refused, stating that he would be willing to attend only outpatient rehabilitation, because the partial hospital program would interfere with his job and his relationship with his girlfriend. The addictionologist believes that outpatient rehabilitation will not be sufficient to treat Jerry's substance abuse.

Reviewer's response: This patient has not yet accepted that he has a significant drug and alcohol problem. He meets the criteria for partial hospital rehabilitation and can be approved for this level of care. He cannot be approved for outpatient rehabilitation, because his lifestyle will render outpatient treatment useless.

It is difficult to say that either side is wrong in this debate about voluntary participation in rehabilitation. The reviewer and the provider are simply making different clinical judgments. Given these differences in judgment, how can you convince a reviewer to approve care for a patient who is not willing to participate in treatment? The best approach is to clearly describe how you will confront your patient's lack of cooperation and what limits you will set on the patient's behavior. You might, for example, state that you will discharge the patient if he or she is still not freely participating in the program after 3 days. Whatever you say, you need to convince the reviewer that the care will not be wasted on an uncooperative patient who is not yet ready for rehabilitation.

What is the goal of treatment?   The last medical necessity criterion for residential rehabilitation is that there be evidence to suggest that the patient will benefit from treatment and remain abstinent. This leads directly to the second question in Table 6–1: What is the goal of treatment and how will you know when you have accomplished it? The goal of all substance abuse rehabilitation is to help the patient remain abstinent outside the program. Yet it is impossible during residential treatment to determine with any certainty whether you have accomplished this goal. In fact, it is much more difficult to determine the progress of rehabilitation than that of detoxification or, for that matter, that of most other psychiatric disorders. If a patient is hospitalized for the treatment of depression or psychosis, the provider expects the target symptoms of these disorders to begin improving before the patient is discharged. In rehabilitation, however, the target symptom is the abuse of a substance. There is no way to determine whether that symptom has improved until after discharge when a patient is faced with temptation and decides not to use the substance.

Many reviewers make determinations of whether a patient will benefit from treatment on the basis of the patient's prior relapses. While reviewing a case with two experienced addictionologists, I argued that the patient did not have a very good prognosis because he had relapsed after three prior courses of rehabilitation. The addictionologists immediately took exception to my statement. One said, "I've been in this business for 20 years and I can't predict whether someone will stay abstinent or not. How can you do it? I've seen a lot of patients who go through three, four, or even five courses of rehabilitation before it finally takes effect." He was right in one sense; I could not predict any more than he could whether the patient would benefit from rehabilitation and remain abstinent. There is no question that some patients who undergo multiple rehabilitations do eventually remain abstinent. Yet it seems logical that the more relapses a patient has, the less likely it is that the next rehabilitation will be successful. Therefore, it seems reasonable after a relapse to expect the patient and provider to present convincing evidence that further rehabilitation will be successful.

This problem was clearly demonstrated in the case of a 43-year-old man I will call Ted. He was admitted for the first time to a 24-hour substance abuse rehabilitation program for treatment of alcohol dependence. Ted underwent a mild alcohol detoxification for 2 days and then entered the rehabilitation component of the program. Two days thereafter, he disappeared from the ward, returning drunk 6 hours later. The program staff allowed him to sober up and continue with rehabilitation treatment. When the practitioner requested additional days of care, the reviewer wanted to know how he could justify continuing to treat the patient in the rehabilitation program after the latter's clandestine drinking episode. The practitioner responded that alcohol dependence was a chronic illness in which the patient often had periodic relapses before attaining a permanent state of sobriety.

The reviewer was not satisfied. "How did you respond to the patient's drinking?" he asked.

"We informed him that it was against the rules of the program," the clinician responded.

"Were there any repercussions for his behavior? How did you confront the issue in treatment?"

"We plugged him back into the rehabilitation program as soon as he was sober."

"How will that stop him from doing the same thing again?"

"We hope he will learn from his behavior and the continuing therapy." The reviewer was still not satisfied. He had several questions about the patient's ability to benefit from the rehabilitation program after his drunken episode. Ted seemed to have little motivation to remain sober. The reviewer expected the clinician and the program staff to focus on the patient's provocative behavior until there was some evidence that the patient understood and accepted responsibility for his behavior. Because this did not occur, the reviewer concluded that the treatment had little likelihood of success, and he recommended that further days of care be denied.

If Ted were your patient, what could you do to convince a reviewer to recommend approval of additional days of care? There are several things. Most important, explain that you and the staff consider the patient's behavior such a significant infraction of the program's rules that you will redesign his treatment plan to focus on this behavior until there is evidence that he understands how serious it is. Argue that the situation actually offers the patient an excellent opportunity to examine, with the help of a supportive staff, the forces that lead him to drink. Describe the criteria you will use to determine whether Ted is responding to the new treatment plan. You might, for example, conclude that the patient is responding if he is able to reflect honestly on the reasons he behaved as he did and suggests steps he might take in the future to avoid such behavior. Finally, explain the circumstances under which you would decide to discharge the patient. You might state that the patient will be discharged in 2 days if there is not clear evidence that he is confronting his behavior and struggling to change it. This should convince the reviewer that you are trying to be as objective as possible and can anticipate the possibility that the patient is not currently treatable.

Suppose instead of having no prior admissions, the patient had two admissions for alcohol abuse in the last 2 years, each followed by a return to drinking within a month of discharge. Now he is presenting for a third admission for rehabilitation. The reviewer is far less likely to recommend approval for another course of treatment for this patient, given his two previous failures. How can you convince the reviewer to give the patient another opportunity for treatment? You might emphasize again that alcohol abuse is a chronic illness associated with multiple relapses. However, if that is all you say, the argument is not likely to be successful. The reviewer will most likely decide that two trials are quite sufficient and that a third admission will not help because the patient is not motivated to stop drinking. You must convince the reviewer that there is something different about this admission that will make it more likely to succeed than previous admissions. Is the patient more motivated for treatment? If so, what is his motivation? Is he about to lose his job or family? Has his drinking led to a significant deterioration in health? Is he having legal problems because of his drinking? You need to explain why you and the patient believe that the patient is now sufficiently motivated to succeed in rehabilitation.

How will you treat the patient?   Once you have demonstrated that your patient fulfills the medical necessity criteria for residential rehabilitation, you need to answer the third question in Table 6–1 and explain how you plan to treat the patient. When you present your treatment plan, it is useful to keep in mind the concerns that many experienced reviewers have about residential rehabilitation programs. If you do so, you can tailor your presentation to respond to these concerns before the reviewer raises them. This will substantially strengthen your argument that the patient will benefit from your residential program.

I hear several common concerns about residential rehabilitation programs from reviewers. First, they argue that some programs have limited effectiveness because they offer cookie-cutter, one-size-fits-all treatment. A 26-year-old unmarried woman receives the same treatment as a 47-year-old married man, even though the two almost certainly have different reasons for drinking and are probably struggling with completely different personal problems. Individuals who have relapsed several times receive the same treatment as those who are receiving rehabilitation for the first time. Even worse, relapsing individuals will often be admitted to the same rehabilitation program they attended before their relapse and be given exactly the same course of treatment that was previously unsuccessful.

Individualized treatment is particularly important for patients who have relapsed. These individuals rarely need to repeat all of the standard lectures and classes on substance abuse. When a reviewer asks how your patient will benefit from another course of residential rehabilitation, explain that the patient will participate in individual and group therapy activities specifically designed for relapsing patients. You need to describe the new treatment plan in some detail, focusing especially on the mechanisms you will use to follow the patient after discharge to prevent another relapse. Tell the reviewer that the sessions will help the patient identify the events that triggered his or her relapse and develop more effective methods of responding to those events in the future. It might be useful to offer a specific example of an event that led to the patient's renewed drinking or use of drugs. The example should be accompanied by a brief explanation of how the issue will be addressed in relapse therapy.

Reviewers are also concerned about programs that are too rigidly structured to respond to a patient's individual needs. By *rigid* they mean that the program requires a patient to stay in treatment for a set period or to complete a specific series of therapeutic steps before discharge. This is not necessarily a problem. Clinicians argue that they are trying to provide a highly structured program for their substance abuse patients because they believe the patients will do better in such an environment. This approach becomes a problem, however, when the clinical staff focuses more on the structure and rules of the program than its therapeutic goals.

One provider was quite candid with me when we discussed the problem of determining an appropriate length of treatment for residential patients. He said, "Residential rehabilitation programs used to be 28 days because that was the duration of the average insurance company's benefit for rehabilitation." Reviewers know this. When they are told that a program has a required length of stay for every patient, they want to hear some clinical justification for the patient's continued stay. If you do have a standard-length program, make sure that you can offer a good reason why it is necessary for your particular patient. Better yet, talk about the patient's current clinical status rather than the need to fit him or her into a standard-length program.

Some rehabilitation programs are more rigid with respect to the therapeutic tasks the patient must accomplish than to the length of stay. One practitioner told a reviewer that her patient could not be discharged after 2 weeks of residential rehabilitation because he had only reached step 5 in their 12-step Alcoholics Anonymous program. She indicated that the patient would be ready for discharge once he had progressed through all 12 steps, but she could not estimate how long that might take. The important issue for the reviewer, however, was not whether the patient had completed all 12 steps but whether he could remain abstinent after discharge to partial hospital or outpatient care. He expected the practitioner to give specific clinical reasons why the patient needed further residential care. When she did not do so, he argued that the patient could continue to progress through the 12-

step program in outpatient Alcoholics Anonymous meetings.

Occasionally, reviewers complain that a program is offering unconventional treatments that seem to them to have questionable therapeutic benefit. Examples of such atypical treatments include equine therapy, rock climbing therapy, and wilderness survival therapy. The issue is not whether such activities will or will not help a patient remain abstinent. Valuable as they may be, these activities are generally not considered to be major modes of treatment supported by the professional community and reimbursed by health insurance. Most insurance plans cover standard, accepted modes of treatment such as individual, group, and family therapy. Reviewers will not argue with you if you provide horseback riding or rock climbing as supplemental activities, so long as they do not replace the established therapies.

Reviewers repeatedly express their concern about residential rehabilitation programs that are staffed mainly with addiction counselors who have limited clinical training. They argue that such paraprofessionals have traditionally provided self-help therapy rather than medical treatment. There is nothing wrong with using drug counselors to treat substance abuse patients. Many counselors have had first-hand experience with alcohol or drug abuse and use that experience to help patients fight their addiction. Yet such programs charge for counseling services as though they were offering medical care, even when there is little active medical intervention or staff supervision. Reviewers believe that if substance abuse treatment is going to be reimbursed as a medical benefit, there should be evidence of active physician involvement in the patient's treatment. A physician should evaluate each patient at the time of admission into the program, periodically see the patient, and document the patient's treatment and progress with a note in the medical record. Medical oversight is particularly important for the evaluation and treatment of individuals with coexisting substance abuse and psychiatric disorders. It takes a great deal of clinical experience to distinguish between a primary psychiatric disorder and changes in mood and thought produced by abuse of drugs.

Medical oversight is important for every residential rehabilitation. A program that is led by a physician and staffed chiefly with certified addiction counselors is rarely considered adequate. Reviewers and insurance companies expect addiction programs to be staffed with a range of highly trained clinicians from several specialties, including nursing, social work, and psychology. Each of these disciplines brings its own approach to treatment. Some insurance plans go further and mandate that individual, group, and family therapy be led by a nurse, social worker, or psychologist with a minimum of a master's degree.

Reviewers and insurance companies also expect to see specific documentation that delineates what transpired in each therapy session and how the patient participated in the session. Although this may seem like a potential breach of confidentiality, there are ways to fulfill the requirements and still protect the patient's privacy. The intent of the regulations is to make sure that patients are actually receiving substantive treatment. Therefore, write your clinical note to fulfill this requirement. Suppose, for example, that a patient states that he drinks when he is angry with his wife because he knows it upsets her. You do not need to write that statement verbatim in your clinical note. Instead you can write, "The patient actively discussed the effect of alcohol on his relationship with his wife." That statement is sufficiently detailed to indicate that the patient participated in a therapeutic encounter, but general enough to hide the specifics of his relationship with his wife.

Determining when a patient in residential rehabilitation is ready for discharge is always a difficult task. Ideally, the decision should be based on a determination of the patient's ability to remain abstinent after discharge. Many clinicians believe that the longer a patient remains in treatment, the better. Reviewers have a somewhat different point of view. They believe that a patient should stay in treatment as long as there are justifiable reasons for him or her to do so. What is or is not a justifiable reason is, of course, open to interpretation. The most convincing arguments for continued stay are based on specific problems in the patient's life, not on substance abuse rehabilitation theory. The reviewer will assess the problems in the context of the patient's current level of care. In one case, for example, a clinician asked for an additional day of residential treatment for a patient because he wanted to explore the possibility that the patient might know or have a personal relationship with another member of her outpatient Alcoholics Anonymous group. The reviewer refused the request because he believed that the issue could be addressed in outpatient therapy and did not require further residential treatment.

What types of problems justify additional days of residential care? They are often related to the patient's interaction with his or her environment. In one such case, an 18-year-old man was admitted to a residential rehabilitation program because he was using cocaine. After several days of individual and group therapy, he began to accept that he had a drug problem. On the fifth day of treatment, he attended family therapy with his parents. During the session, the patient and his father got into a violent argument and the patient threw his can of soda against the wall, splattering his father with the contents. The parents refused to take the patient home with them when he was discharged, because of his temper and because they were afraid he would have a bad influence on his younger brother and sister. The patient had nowhere else to go. The staff believed that he was less likely to relapse if he returned home after discharge. Additional time was requested for more family sessions to help the patient settle some of his differences with his father. The reviewer approved 3 additional days with the understanding that the staff would work on alternative discharge plans in case the family disputes could not be resolved.

Additional days of residential care may also be justified if the clinical staff identify a significant comorbid disorder that requires treatment. That was the case for a 26-year-old unemployed woman who abused heroin. After 4 days of rehabilitation, her clinician began to suspect that she was significantly depressed and had been so as an adolescent, before she began using heroin. The clinician asked for approval of additional days of rehabilitation to have the patient evaluated by a psychiatrist and, if necessary, begin taking antidepressant medication. He told the reviewer that it would be difficult to treat the patient's heroin abuse without addressing the depression. A psychiatric consultation was scheduled for the next day. When the reviewer asked why the consultation had to be done while the patient was in the residential program, the clinician argued that it would take longer to arrange an outpatient appointment and the patient might relapse during the wait. In addition, if the patient needed antidepressant medication, the staff wanted to see how she tolerated it for at least a day. He argued further that the patient was far more likely to remain abstinent if her depression was treated. The reviewer approved 1 more day of residential care for the psychiatric evaluation and subsequently approved another 2 days to begin treatment with antidepressant medication.

Patients with comorbid disorders present another treatment problem. If the patient requires hospitalization, the clinician often must decide between admitting the patient to an inpatient psychiatric ward and admitting him or her to an inpatient substance abuse rehabilitation unit. Unfortunately, many psychiatric services do not offer substantive drug or alcohol rehabilitation treatment. Similarly, many rehabilitation units do not provide effective psychiatric care. Therefore, if you decide to admit a patient with a dual diagnosis to either type of service, you will have to convince the reviewer that your patient will receive the full range of care he or she needs (see Case 6–5).

Case 6–5: Nicholas is suicidal when drunk

Clinical presentation: Nicholas is a 52-year-old man who arrived at the emergency department late one evening stating that he was going to kill himself. His blood alcohol level was 0.36. Nicholas was treated in the emergency department with intravenous fluids, vitamins, and Librium. The next morning, he was sober and medically stable and denied wanting to kill himself. The emergency physician wanted to admit him to the psychiatric unit for treatment of depression and suicidal ideation.

Reviewer's response: Why does the physician want to admit the patient to a psychiatric unit? He is no longer suicidal. His main problem appears to be his alcohol abuse. It will be difficult to assess his depression accurately until his alcohol abuse has been addressed. It would make sense to admit him to an alcohol rehabilitation program where his depression could also be evaluated. He won't receive sufficient substance abuse treatment in a standard psychiatric unit.

How will you maintain the patient's abstinence after discharge?   The main goal of residential rehabilitation is to significantly increase the likelihood that a patient will remain abstinent after discharge from the program. Most reviewers believe that the most effective way of doing this is to actively prepare the patient for his or her environment and to prepare the environment for the patient. When I say prepare the patient for his or her environment, I mean help the patient identify the circumstances in his or her life outside the program that drive the patient to abuse drugs or alcohol, and teach him or her how to avoid these circumstances or confront them more effectively. Preparing the environment, on the other hand, means directly intervening to change some of the conditions in the patient's life outside the program that facilitate his or her drug or alcohol abuse.

The role of the environment in maintaining a patient's addiction is graphically demonstrated in the case of Jean, a 25-year-old single, employed woman who was addicted to cocaine. Two months before her admission to a residential rehabilitation program, she was evicted from her apartment for failing to pay the rent. Jean later told her substance abuse counselor that she had no money for the rent because she spent her paycheck on cocaine as soon as she received it. After the eviction, Jean moved to a fleabag hotel, paying for her room on a day-to-day basis, scrounging money where she could.

It was obvious to the entire rehabilitation team that even with ongoing outpatient therapy and Narcotics Anonymous meetings, Jean would probably start using cocaine again if she returned to the run-down hotel where she lived. The team needed to prepare the environment for Jean by finding her a new living arrangement where she would not be so isolated. As the rehabilitation progressed, the social worker responsible for helping Jean make discharge plans suggested that she move back home with her mother. This was not feasible, because Jean's mother was a carnival sideshow belly dancer who was on the road much of the year. After several telephone calls, the social worker finally made arrangements for Jean to move in with her mother's cousin. Jean agreed to pay the woman for her room and board. The rehabilitation team also realized that they needed to prepare Jean for her new environment by having someone control her paycheck and make sure she did not spend it on cocaine as soon as she received it. They eventually convinced her to have the paycheck managed by her cousin, who agreed to pay her bills.

It is often the small details and problems of life, those the patient may not spontaneously speak of, that make a difference between the ability and the inability to remain abstinent. One 32-year-old man, for example, revealed that his wife and mother-in-law were social drinkers who refused to stop drinking over holidays despite the patient's problems with alcohol. He often felt compelled to join them even though he subsequently drank to excess. Once the problem was identified in therapy, he learned to spend his time at Alcoholics Anonymous meetings when his family was drinking during the holidays. That might seem like an obvious solution, but it had not occurred to the patient until he discussed the issue in detail with his therapist. Another patient, confronted with the fact that she did not attend Alcoholics Anonymous meetings after discharge from a prior rehabilitation program, stated that she felt uncomfortable with the spirituality inherent in Alcoholics Anonymous meetings. When staff members became aware of this problem, they referred her to a modified program with less spiritual emphasis. Again, the solution to this patient's problem appeared obvious only in retrospect.

Once a patient is admitted to a residential rehabilitation program, a reviewer will begin to press you to explain why the patient needs to continue in the program. You may feel that the reviewer is not giving you the time to treat the patient. But what the reviewer is really doing is challenging you to defend your decision to admit and keep the patient in the residential program. Your job is to identify the specific problems that make it difficult for the patient to remain abstinent, and then develop a reasonable treatment plan that addresses each problem. Most reviewers will continue to approve care if the problems you identify seem relevant to the patient's residential treatment and you are actively working to resolve them.

Suggested Reading

Barnes HN, Samet JH: Brief interventions with substance-abusing patients. Med Clin North Am 81:867–879, 1997

Bukstein O: Practice parameters for the assessment and treatment of children and adolescents with substance use disorders. American Academy of Child and Adolescent Psychiatry. J Am Acad Child Adolesc Psychiatry 36:140S–156S, 1997

Bukstein O: Summary of the practice parameters for the assessment and treatment of children and adolescents with substance use disorders. J Am Acad Child Adolesc Psychiatry 37:122–126, 1998

Chappel JN, DuPont RL: Twelve-step and mutual-help programs for addictive disorders. Psychiatr Clin North Am 22:425–446, 1999

Fishman M, Bruner A, Adger H: Substance abuse among children and adolescents. Pediatr Rev 18:394–403, 1997

Francis E, Hughes P, Schinka J: Improving cost-effectiveness in a substance abuse treatment program. Psychiatr Serv 50:633–635, 1999

Friedmann PD, Saitz R, Samet JH: Management of adults recovering from alcohol or other drug problems: relapse prevention in primary care. JAMA 279:1227–1231, 1998

Goldsmith RJ: Overview of psychiatric comorbidity: practical and theoretic considerations. Psychiatr Clin North Am 22:331–349, 1999

Grant B: Barriers to alcoholism treatment: reasons for not seeking treatment in a general population sample. J Stud Alcohol 58:365–371, 1997

Harrison PA, Asche SE: Comparison of substance abuse treatment outcomes for inpatients and outpatients. J Subst Abuse Treat 17:207–220, 1999

Hoff RA, Rosenheck RA: The cost of treating substance abuse patients with and without comorbid psychiatric disorders. Psychiatr Serv 50:1309–1315, 1999

Indications for management and referral of patients involved in substance abuse. American Academy of Pediatrics. Pediatrics 106:143–48, 2000

Kaufman E: Diagnosis and treatment of drug and alcohol abuse in women. Am J Obstet Gynecol 174:21–27, 1996

Larson MJ, Samet JH, McCarty D: Managed care of substance abuse disorders: implications for generalist physicians. Med Clin North Am 81:1053–1069, 1997

Miller NS, Flaherty JA: Effectiveness of coerced addiction treatment (alternative consequences): a review of the clinical literature. J Subst Abuse Treat 18:9–16, 2000

Miller NS, Gold MS: Management of withdrawal syndromes and relapse prevention in drug and alcohol dependence. Am Fam Physician 58:139–146, 1998

Nunes EV, Deliyannides D, Donovan S, et al: The management of treatment resistance in depressed patients with substance abuse disorders. Psychiatr Clin North Am 19:311–327, 1996

Olmedo R, Hoffman RS: Withdrawal syndromes. Emerg Med Clin North Am 18:273–288, 2000

Ross SM, Chappel JN: Substance use disorders: difficulties in diagnosis. Psychiatr Clin North Am 21:803–828, 1998

Rumpf HJ, Hapke U, Meyer C, et al: Motivation to change drinking behavior: comparison of alcohol-dependent individuals in a general hospital and a general population sample. Gen Hosp Psychiatry 21:348–353, 1999

Samet JH, O'Connor PG: Alcohol abusers in primary care: readiness to change behavior. Am J Med 105:302–306, 1998

Satel SL: What should we expect from drug abusers (editorial)? Psychiatr Serv 50:861, 1999

Shepard DS, Larson MJ, Hoffmann NG: Cost-effectiveness of substance abuse services: implications for public policy. Psychiatr Clin North Am 22:385–400, 1999

Shiffman S: Comments on craving. Addiction 95 (suppl 2):S171–S175, 2000

Weisner C, Mertens J, Parthasarathy S, et al: The outcome and cost of alcohol and drug treatment in an HMO: day hospital versus traditional outpatient regimens. Health Serv Res 35:791–812, 2000

CHAPTER 7

Fundamentals of Clinical Documentation

No matter how effectively you argue your patient's case in a concurrent review, you will still have to support your clinical decisions with detailed documentation in the patient's medical record. Managed care and insurance companies routinely conduct retrospective reviews of medical records after a patient has been discharged, to verify that the patient's care met the required medical necessity criteria. In a retrospective review, unlike a concurrent review, there is no overt interference in the doctor–patient relationship, no denial of care, and no restriction on the physician's decision making with regard to the patient's treatment. Concurrent and retrospective reviews also differ in the type and source of information they use. A concurrent review is based on an oral description of the patient's clinical condition at one particular point in time, given by a single clinician. The retrospective review, on the other hand, is based on a detailed written record of the patient's treatment during an entire episode of illness, with contributions from multiple clinicians.

Superficially, it may seem that the retrospective review is a kinder, gentler, and less intrusive process for patients, providers, and health care facilities. That is only partially true. Although the retrospective review has less direct impact on the patient than the concurrent review does, it can have even more impact on the hospital and provider, because it is a far more detailed scrutiny of the patient's care. Every decision made by the physician, and every service provided by the treatment team, is examined to determine whether it was appropriate and necessary. The insurance company may withhold payment to the facility and provider for all services that are judged inappropriate or unnecessary for the patient's care.

You may think, after reading this description, that you have even less control over your clinical practice under the retrospective review process than you do under the concurrent review process. That is not necessarily true. Your success in a retrospective review depends on the type of information you document in your patient's medical record, and how you document it. Clinicians often mistakenly assume that reviewers use the same information that they themselves use to arrive at decisions about the necessity and appropriateness of a patient's care. Medical record reviewers, however, have learned that much of the information in any given medical record is irrelevant for the work they are trying to do.

Why is there such a discrepancy between the information requirements of providers and those of reviewers? The main reason is that the two groups have different goals. Clinicians believe that everything they learn about a patient is potentially useful in the patient's treatment. If a clinician discovers that his severely depressed patient's father died at age 40 and that the patient will be 40 in 2 months, he will document this information in the patient's clinical record and focus on it in treatment. Reviewers, on the other hand, are looking for very specific information that either justifies or does not justify a patient's admission to or continuing stay in the treatment program. The information a reviewer requires is stipulated in the medical necessity criteria. He or she is not interested in the depressed patient's family history. The reviewer is concerned about the severity of the patient's depression, his potential for suicide, and his ability to care for himself out of the hospital. If you clearly supply this information in the patient's record, there is a much higher likelihood that the reviewer will approve your patient's care. The most efficient way to do this is to make sure that you include the information the reviewer needs in your standard clinical notes.

When you write a note in a patient's clinical record, organize it to answer the four questions I discussed in Chapters 4, 5, and 6: Why does the patient need the level of care you are requesting now? What are you trying to accomplish with the care and how will you know when you have accomplished it? How will you treat the patient? What are you planning to do with the patient after discharge? When you answer these questions in writing, you need to be just as specific as you are during a telephone discussion with a reviewer. There is, however, a significant difference between orally presenting a case and documenting information in the patient's chart. When you speak to the reviewer, he or she can ask questions for clarification. When you write notes in the chart, you must anticipate the reviewer's questions and discuss them in an organized manner so that the reviewer can follow your thoughts about the patient's treatment as it evolved (Table 7–1).

The reviewer can trace the evolution of treatment only if your notes are

---

Table 7-1.   Keys to effective documentation

- **Conceptualize your case:** Gather clinical information and synthesize it into a comprehensive, coherent narrative of the patient's illness that identifies the patient's problems, provides a diagnosis, and specifies the goals, methods, and expected outcome of treatment.

- **Write convincing notes:** The patient's record as a whole and all its individual entries should convey a sense of consistency and truth.

- **Explain inconsistencies:** Read the notes that other clinicians have written in the patient's clinical record and explain any inconsistencies between your observations and theirs.

- **Use accepted terminology:** Avoid nonstandard terms and phrases. Create a glossary of acceptable terms and abbreviations for your facility. Include this glossary with each chart sent for review.

- **Write legibly:** Make sure your handwriting is legible, or dictate your notes and then proofread and sign the transcribed copy. In every patient record, include a signature page with examples of each clinician's signature next to his or her typed name.

---

timely and are easily identified within the medical record. Do not make the mistake that one psychiatrist did. He dictated five progress notes at the end of 1 week and placed the transcribed notes, all typed on the same page, into the medical record the following Monday. The reviewer interpreted this as evidence that the psychiatrist was neither giving significant direction to the treatment team nor providing accurate, timely documentation of the patient's clinical status and response to treatment. Remember, you are trying to establish credibility with a reviewer. Once you have done that, he or she will be willing to give you some latitude in caring for the patient because the reviewer believes that you are a competent and concerned clinician. You can establish a great deal of credibility by writing timely, legible notes that clearly document your clinical observations, conclusions, and decisions.

Conceptualize Your Case

When a reviewer examines a medical record, he or she looks first to see whether the patient's clinician has adequately conceptualized the case. By this I mean that the clinician has gathered important information about the patient and synthesized that information into a comprehensive, coherent narrative of the patient's illness that clearly identifies the patient's clinical problems, presents a reasonable diagnosis, and specifies the goals, methods, and potential outcome of treatment in enough detail for the reviewer to assess whether the patient is receiving appropriate care. The active synthesis of clinical information is the crucial intellectual element that defines the role of the clinician leading the treatment team. That clinician may be a psychiatrist, psychologist, social worker, or nurse. If the patient has a psychiatrist, however, most reviewers will assume that the psychiatrist is the leader of the clinical team, because physicians have traditionally been given the ultimate responsibility for care of the patient. As a physician, the surest way to invite close scrutiny of your cases is to avoid accepting the clinical leadership role. The best way to deflect that scrutiny is to clearly conceptualize each case in writing and document your ongoing observations, conclusions, and decisions so that they can guide the clinical staff throughout the patient's treatment. If a reviewer finds evidence of such active, ongoing conceptualization, he or she is generally less apt to intently scrutinize the patient's chart.

When there is no active clinical leadership, treatment may seem fragmented, drifting from day to day without clearly stated goals or end points. Each clinician on the team comments on his or her specific interaction with the patient, but there is little evidence that someone is assessing the overall progress of the patient's treatment or making sense of seeming contradictions. Take, for example, the case of George, a 29-year-old man who was admitted to the hospital with an acute manic episode. Six days later, a group therapist wrote, "George was calmer and more appropriate in group this morning." That same day, a nurse observed in her shift report, "The patient was disruptive at lunch and couldn't sit still. He paced the halls this afternoon." The occupational therapist commented, "George worked on his project this afternoon and made more progress than usual." Finally, the psychiatrist's note stated, "Patient unchanged. Lithium level 0.6 mEq/L. Continue lithium 300 mg tid." When a reviewer sees these seeming contradictions, he or she automatically begins to examine the medical record for evidence of other problems with care. Inevitably, the reviewer finds them. Perhaps worse, if the contradictions are not put into perspective, the reviewer will choose whatever documentation is needed to support his or her argument that the patient does not require additional care.

Clinical leadership and conceptualization are not new ideas, yet when I raised these issues with one physician during a review, he replied, "I couldn't do that. I would have to write a one-page progress note every time I saw the patient to fulfill your requirements." Unfortunately, he drew the wrong conclusion from my statements. What is important is not the length of the note but its organization and content. In Mr. B's case, someone has to explain the seeming discrepancies in a clinically meaningful way and set the course for continuing care. A good clinician can summarize the important elements of the case in a few well-chosen words:

> Reports by various clinical staff members indicate that the patient's symptoms are waxing and waning throughout the day. See today's notes from group therapy 10:00 A.M. and OT [occupational therapy] 4:30 P.M., also afternoon nursing report. I met with the patient at 5:30 P.M. He seemed marginally calmer than yesterday, but his speech remained rapid, he still had some grandiose financial plans, and he paced the room while we spoke. The patient is beginning to respond to his lithium. I will look for more consistent evidence that his symptoms are under control before considering discharge. In the meantime, we will continue arranging his follow-up outpatient care. A family meeting is scheduled for tomorrow.

Provide Convincing Documentation

What makes clinical documentation convincing? People who write fiction speak about verisimilitude. They mean by that term that the story has the appearance or semblance of truth. The same word can be used in reference to clinical documentation. A patient's record has verisimilitude when the document as a whole, as well as the individual observations, conclusions, and decisions it contains, makes sense. Reviewers are sensitive to any incongruity that casts doubt on the verisimilitude of the documentation and, by extrapolation, the quality of care.

Just such a problem was evident in the case of an inpatient who was placed on 15-minute checks because her psychiatrist was concerned about her potential for self-destructive behavior. The reviewer noticed that the patient had been missing from the ward for 3 hours during one nursing shift. He wondered how this could have happened if the patient was being watched so closely. When he examined the checklist that documented the nurses' 15-minute observations of the patient, it appeared to him that all the observations for the shift in question had been initialed by the same nurse at the same time. He concluded, correctly or incorrectly, that the nurse had never actually made the individual 15-minute observations, because it would have been impossible to do so if the patient was not on the ward. This single discrepancy was sufficient to raise questions about the validity of the patient's entire medical record.

Subtle and not so subtle incongruities appear in many clinical charts. Most patients, for example, respond to successful treatment with gradual improvement. Therefore, it does not make much sense to the reviewer if there are notes indicating that a patient is acutely psychotic or suicidal for 10 days and then is suddenly discharged, with the symptoms resolved, on the eleventh day. Occasionally, patients do have a dramatic response to treatment, but this is not usually true. The main reason practitioners emphasize the severity of a patient's illness until the moment before discharge is that they are concerned that if the patient begins to show improvement, the insurance company will deny further days of care. Although this is a realistic concern, it is better to document what you learn from the patient each day so that your successive notes provide a cogent and believable picture of the patient's response to treatment. Use this information as the basis of your argument to justify the patient's continuing hospitalization.

The issue of when to discharge a patient from inpatient care is always an area of contention between practitioners and reviewers. The patient cannot stay in the hospital indefinitely. At some point during treatment, a decision must be made to discharge the patient. The decision is most difficult with patients who are psychotic, express suicidal ideation, or threaten violence. In retrospective reviews, I often ask providers how they make the decision to discharge a suicidal patient. In many cases, the medical record documents that the patient has denied suicidal ideation several times, yet is still hospitalized. "At what point," I ask, "do you believe the patient's denials and discharge him or her?" Most practitioners have difficulty answering this question. They often respond that after years of experience, they have developed something of a clinical sixth sense that helps them decide whether the patient is still truly suicidal. The details and rationale for this decision, however, are rarely documented in the physician's clinical note, and as a result, the decision seems random. If you wish to have your decisions appear logical, you must give some thought to how you make the decision to discharge such a patient, and communicate the rationale for the decision in your progress note. It is not sufficient to state your opinion that the patient is no longer suicidal. You must explain why you now believe the patient's denials, when you ignored them in the past.

One common mistake that clinicians often make is to identify a clinical problem, such as suicidal ideation, but never focus on it again in the clinical documentation. If a patient is hospitalized mainly because his or her thinking is so disorganized that the patient is a danger to self, you should write a note every day documenting his or her thought processes. If a symptom is serious enough to justify a patient's hospitalization, the reviewer will expect that the symptom will be closely monitored throughout the patient's stay in the hospital. If it is not monitored closely, the reviewer may conclude that it was not a very serious problem to begin with and that the patient probably did not meet the medical necessity criteria for admission.

It does no good to make accurate observations and reasonable clinical decisions if you cannot communicate them in a coherent progress note to other staff members as well as reviewers. When you write a note, your observations, interpretations, and conclusions should follow one another in a logical sequence, culminating in a defensible treatment decision. This rule may seem so obvious that it does not bear comment, yet it is often neglected. Convoluted, illogical, or incoherent notes are far too common in routine clinical records. Consider this statement written in a patient's chart: "The fact that the patient's attendance in the program was erratic proves that he needed to be there." Following this line of circular reasoning, one would have to conclude that if the patient attended the program, he would not need it. It would have been far better if the physician had asked the patient about his absences and documented his response with a statement such as "I discussed the patient's erratic attendance with him and he stated that he has difficulty getting to the program and doesn't feel he is receiving any benefit from it." A reviewer reading the latter statement would realize that the physician was trying to address the patient's specific resistance to treatment, rather than trying to justify it on dubious theoretical grounds.

Sometimes a note is so complicated, with so many conditions and qualifications, that after several readings it is still difficult to understand. One clinician wrote, "The patient is competent to be able to determine if she wants to let anybody know if she is suicidal or not." Is the clinician concerned about the patient's mental competence, her ability to determine her own wishes, her willingness to tell someone when she feels suicidal, or her current suicidal intent? Presumably, the most important question is whether the patient will inform another person when she feels suicidal. The clinician might have written instead: "The patient agreed to inform another person if she feels suicidal." The most useful clinical notes are constructed with simple sentences that contain one or two thoughts. People may enjoy being challenged by complicated literary sentences in a novel, but in a clinical report they want to get to the point as quickly and unambiguously as possible. Therefore, keep your progress notes and sentences short and focused on the main topic.

Ambiguous clinical notes are as bad as those that are too complicated. Consider the following: "The patient will be placed on unpredictable precautions" and "The patient described racing clouds." In the first sentence, it is difficult to determine whether the patient or the precautions are unpredictable. Presumably, the clinician thinks the patient is unpredictable and needs to be closely watched. Unfortunately, the word *unpredictable* is too ambiguous. How is the patient unpredictable? Is he violent, self-destructive, impulsive, or overly amorous? One cannot tell from the note. Would it not make more sense to specify the unpredictable acts?

The second note is ambiguous because it is incomplete. Did the patient describe a visual hallucination or illusion? Was she offering a poetic image? Could the clinician mean "racing thoughts"? It is impossible to determine what this sentence means without further elaboration. The clinician could have written: "The patient reported seeing clouds racing across the sky. This phenomenon was not evident to anyone speaking to her at the time" or "The patient reported seeing clouds racing across the ceiling of her room at night." Both elaborations make it clear that the patient was experiencing some type of perceptual distortion.

The main problem with all of these confusing progress notes is that they convey little useful information about the patient's clinical condition. Beyond that, they raise questions about the credibility of the clinicians who wrote them. A reviewer reading one of these notes will almost certainly wonder about the physician's clinical judgment and ability to treat the patient. In response, the reviewer will usually ignore the illogical note and scrutinize the case even more closely for inconsistencies. Unfortunately, clinical credibility once lost is difficult to regain.

Provide Consistent Information

The most common reason reviewers deny reimbursement in a retrospective review is that they detect significant inconsistencies in the information written in the patient's medical record. These inconsistencies take several forms. In one, the physician's oral report of the patient's medical status, provided to the reviewer during the concurrent review, is not adequately substantiated by information in the medical record. For example, a physician may tell a reviewer over the telephone that his patient is acutely suicidal and planned to kill herself with an overdose on the night of admission. He may supply all the details of a complete suicide evaluation and convince the reviewer that the patient is truly a danger to herself. The admitting note in the chart, however, may simply state: "The patient has suicidal ideation." Because this documentation does not, by itself, adequately demonstrate the need for immediate hospitalization, and because the individual who performs the retrospective review may not have access to the detailed information from the original telephone conversation, the reviewer may deny payment for the hospitalization. To forestall this possibility, make sure you document the details of your telephone conversation with the first reviewer in the patient's medical record. Remember, the chart is a legal document and the final repository of information on the patient's illness and treatment. The oral review is merely a convenience, a means of responding to the reviewer's concerns and clarifying the patient's condition. It must be documented to become part of the patient's permanent record.

In another type of inconsistency, the physician documents the same clinical details he or she orally presented to the reviewer, but these details are not substantiated by notes and reports from other staff members. For example, a physician may repeatedly state in his progress notes that the patient is still disorganized, psychotic, or potentially violent. At the same time, notes from other staff members may indicate that the patient was able to adequately attend to her activities of daily life, denied hallucinations, had no obvious thought disorder, and was cooperative with staff and other patients. The reviewer must try to reconcile these inconsistencies. Sometimes this is easy. If, for example, the patient's illness is characterized by waxing and waning symptoms and erratic behavior, it makes sense that different clinicians would see different aspects of the illness at different times. Many psychiatric symptoms fluctuate in intensity and duration. Some patients cycle through feelings of rage or suicidal ideation several times a day. If this is the case, however, the physician should comment in the progress note on the fluctuating nature of the patient's illness—not to satisfy the reviewer but to alert the other members of the clinical team to the problem. If a reviewer sees multiple inconsistencies in the medical record that are not explained by the physician, he or she is likely to conclude that the nursing staff, psychologists, and social workers, who generally spend more time with the patient than the physician does, are providing the more accurate account of the patient's illness.

Although it is easy to understand how various staff members can observe different aspects of the patient's behavior over time, it is more difficult to accept ongoing discrepancies in the patient's history. In one case, a physician's admission note stated that the patient reported suicidal ideation but had made no prior suicide attempt. A day later, a nurse wrote in the chart that the week before admission, the patient had attempted suicide by jumping out of a second-story window. This difference is not a problem if it is addressed and documented in the record. The staff should question the patient to try to resolve the different reports. In the process, they may discover additional important information about the patient's clinical condition. The patient might have felt too ashamed at the time of admission to tell the physician about his prior suicide attempt. Once on the psychiatric ward, he might have felt more comfortable talking to the nurse. The most important thing is not the discrepancy but how it is handled by the staff. If it is not addressed in the patient's medical record, the reviewer will assume that staff members do not read each other's notes and that there is little coordination of care. If, on the other hand, the reviewer sees a note discussing the discrepancy, he or she will probably conclude that the patient is receiving high-quality care. Small details like this positively influence a reviewer's attitude toward staff and a facility. This tends to make him or her less critical during subsequent reviews.

Sometimes inconsistencies arise from policies within a facility. To save time, one hospital adopted an electronic medical record that reprinted several paragraphs from the admission summary as part of the discharge summary. This produced a problem for one physician when he reported, in his admission note, that an alcohol-dependent patient had stated that no one else in the family had problems with alcohol. On the second day, the patient told the social worker that all his brothers and sisters were alcoholic. Despite this difference, the incorrect information from the admission summary was reprinted as part of the discharge summary. The reviewer who discovered this discrepancy began to question the physician's and staff's credibility. Such errors may seem trivial, but they raise questions about communication between various staff members caring for the patient and about the overall quality of care. Perhaps worse, they often drive the reviewer to scrutinize the medical record far more closely than if he or she had not detected a discrepancy.

More disturbing than an inconsistency in the medical record due to a careless clerical error is a situation in which a patient's treatment is inconsistent with his or her clinical condition. In one case, a patient was described as confused, disoriented, and incontinent of urine and stool. Yet the patient's treatment plan stated that he would be treated with daily individual and group psychotherapy. The staff might argue that this was an innocent mistake. Yet at the least, it raises questions about the relevance of the written documentation, because no one detected and corrected the inconsistency. At the worst, it suggests a significant problem with the quality and appropriateness of care, if the clinicians involved believed that such psychotherapy was appropriate for the patient.

A similar type of inconsistency arose when a facility requested authorization to admit a patient from the emergency department after she took an overdose of a few analgesic pills. The facility was initially informed that the patient had no insurance benefits. The hospital psychiatrist conducting the intake interview spoke with the patient, concluded that she did not meet criteria for admission because she was no longer suicidal, and decided not to admit the patient. Shortly thereafter, the facility discovered that the patient did have insurance benefits. A subsequent note from the psychiatrist stated that the patient was suicidal, and she was admitted. To the reviewer, it appeared that the decision to admit was based solely on the patient's insurance status. This glaring discrepancy could have been partly resolved if the psychiatrist had explained, in his evaluation, why he disagreed with the original assessment and decided to admit the patient.

One final type of inconsistency relates to documentation of the clinical services provided to the patient. Many insurance companies require clinicians and facilities to provide specific services to their patients. They may stipulate, for example, that a patient in a substance abuse rehabilitation unit attend two full 90-minute group therapy sessions each day unless there is a specific reason, documented in the medical record, that the patient cannot attend the entire session. Furthermore, they may demand that the beginning and ending times of the session, the credentials of the group leaders, general details of the group discussion, and some assessment of the patient's participation in the group be recorded in the medical record. Although these demands for documentation may seem excessive, they developed in response to programs that defined therapeutic groups so loosely that sessions were often no more than brief, casual discussions between patients and staff members who were not adequately trained to conduct true group therapy sessions. Reviewers are especially quick to detect and question subtle discrepancies in a patient's schedule of activities. In one case, several days of nurses' notes for a patient, written before a scheduled morning group began, stated that the patient would attend group therapy from 10:30 to 11:30 A.M. The group notes, however, stated that the patient was scheduled for group therapy from 10:30 A.M. to 12:00 P.M. but could tolerate only 60 minutes. To the reviewer, it appeared that the clinician's intent from the beginning was to provide 60 minutes of group therapy. If that was not so, why would the nurses have written in advance that the patient would have only an hour of group therapy? It would have been far better if the nurses had explained, in advance, that the patient could tolerate only 1 hour of group therapy and if they had discussed how the staff were going to respond to the patient's problem.

Inconsistencies appear in every medical record. Some are trivial mistakes and misunderstandings, but others reveal important problems in the delivery of clinical care. These may be unintentional or intentional. Reviewers are detectives, alert for inconsistencies because they reveal problems with the quality and appropriateness of care. Once a significant inconsistency is detected, it is the responsibility of the clinician and facility to explain it to the reviewer's satisfaction. If this is not done, the credibility of the clinician and facility suffers.

Write Legibly and Use Accepted Terminology

If you want to increase the likelihood that a reviewer will approve your patient's care, you must write legibly and use standard clinical terminology. Although everyone laughs at the illegibility of physician handwriting, it represents a serious problem. If the physician is the leader of the medical team, his or her notes and orders must be readable to minimize errors and guide the team in treating the patient. Unfortunately, the physician's handwriting is illegible in at least one-third of the medical charts that I review.

Reviewers have a variety of responses to illegible physician notes—none of them positive. Some equate illegible notes with disorganized thinking and substandard clinical care. Others conclude that the physician was rushed when he or she wrote the note and surmise that the physician must be just as rushed, and is potentially careless, when performing clinical duties. Still others become suspicious when they see such notes, and they assume that the physician is trying to hide something. Most reviewers initially try to read illegible notes. If they have too much difficulty, they disregard the notes and gather the information for their review from other entries in the record. This means that the observations and conclusions of the physician—the one person who is ultimately responsible for the patient—are not used in determining the quality and appropriateness of care. Perhaps worse, the reviewer is often left with a feeling that the patient is receiving poor care, and the reviewer looks for additional information to verify that impression. Therefore, it is to your advantage to make sure that the reviewer can read and understand your documentation. If you have illegible handwriting, dictate your progress notes each day, have them transcribed, place them in the medical record, and sign and date them. Including the time of the observations is also useful.

Whereas illegible handwriting may suggest that you are disorganized, rushed, or trying to hide something, unconventional diagnoses (major depression, first episode, chronic; repressive disorder; psychothymia; judgment disorder, depressed; alcohol recovery stenosis), pseudosymptoms (polycystic thought processes, incohesive speech, mitral wall prolapse, sudden death syndrome, bilateral dentures, speech depravation), and ludicrous phrases ("consider mood stabilizers such as Halibut") convey the impression that you are clinically illiterate or, at the least, that you are careless and never proofread what you have written. Standard diagnoses and clinical descriptions are part of the common language used in the mental health professions. You use them so that other clinicians will understand what you are saying about a patient. When you use idiosyncratic terminology, you prevent this process of communication and leave other clinicians wondering what you are trying to say. One reviewer recently reported just such a problem. While reading the notes of a nurse who was caring for a patient whose medical record he was reviewing, he encountered the following phrase several times: "There is no evidence of 'S.'" It took a while for him to realize that she was probably referring to suicide—although she made no distinction between suicidal ideation and suicide intent. When the reviewer described the abbreviation to the medical director of the facility, he seemed surprised, a reaction that made the reviewer wonder whether the director ever read the medical records. One way to manage the use of such idiosyncratic terms is to create a glossary of accepted medical abbreviations for your facility. If you do this, make sure to include a copy of the glossary with each medical record you send for review.

Suggested Reading

Dwyer J, Shih A: The ethics of tailoring the patient's chart. Psychiatr Serv 49:1309–1312, 1998

Eisen SV: Clinical status: charting for outcomes in behavioral health. Psychiatr Clin North Am 23:347–361, 2000

Keefe RH, Hall ML: Private practitioners' documentation of outpatient psychiatric treatment: questioning managed care. J Behav Health Serv Res 26:151–170, 1999

Kightlinger R: Sloppy records—the kiss of death for a malpractice defense. Med Econ 76:166–168, 171–172, 174, 1999

CHAPTER 8

Documenting an Individual Patient's Care

Clinical documentation should reflect the individuality of each patient. This is an obvious rule, but it bears discussion because many practitioners develop comfortable, general phrases that they habitually use from one clinical note and patient to another. One physician ended each progress note with the statement "Insight-oriented and cognitive-behavioral therapy were provided to the patient in daily individual therapy sessions." There was no elaboration of how the therapy was conducted, nor was there explanation of what topics were discussed or what the patient gained from treatment. Another clinician reported: "The patient was provided with a safe and stable environment." What does that mean? Would any clinician knowingly admit a patient to an unsafe and unstable environment? What information does the note convey about the patient and the patient's treatment? The statement is more window dressing than substance. It is like writing a note stating "The patient was admitted to be treated." There is not enough clinical detail in any of these examples to convince a reviewer that individualized services were provided to the patient.

Assessments of a patient's response to treatment are often equally generic. Providers treating patients commonly write phrases such as "He is improving." Most reviewers would consider the phrase far too general to use in a progress note without indicating how the patient's specific signs and symptoms were improving. Instead, you might write: "The patient's mental status is improving. Today at 10:00 A.M. he was oriented to person, place, and time. He was also able to correctly do single-digit subtraction in his head." Even a statement such as "She is less depressed" is too generic. A reviewer will have

Table 8-1. Keys to documenting an individual patient's care for review

- Treat each patient as an individual in your documentation.

- Do not use generic or stock phrases to describe a patient's clinical condition, treatment, or goals for treatment.

- Avoid using detailed, overly elaborate checklists to record clinical information. Most clinicians and reviewers find them difficult to read.

- Create brief, simple, hybrid forms that include the most important clinical details in checklist format and allow room for narrative descriptions. Fill them out consistently.

- Write enough meaningful clinical details in your notes to justify your diagnosis, conclusions, and decisions, but do not include personal information that is irrelevant to the treatment and may compromise your patient.

- Provide the information the reviewer needs in your documentation, even if you disagree with the reviewer about what information is important.

several questions about the patient's depression. During what period was the patient less depressed? How was the degree of depression determined? Did the patient state she was less depressed? Was she more physically active? Did she feel less hopeless? You need to be more specific so that the reviewer can distinguish this depressed patient from another (Table 8–1).

The use of some stock phrases is probably unavoidable. It is very difficult to provide an endless stream of individualized, creative descriptions of patients and clinical services. Nevertheless, when every progress note and treatment plan is filled with general, superficial comments, very little information is communicated to the reader. In fact, such notes raise questions about whether the clinician actually saw the patient and spoke to him or her. You might consider the use of these stock phrases acceptable given the increasing volume of patients that you are forced to treat. Unfortunately, I do not think such use can be so easily dismissed. Stock phrases suggest to a reviewer that you have a superficial understanding of the clinical details of the patient's illness. Consider the extreme example of a psychiatrist who used the same phrase in reporting on the mental status examinations of different patients. In each patient's chart, he reported that the patient interpreted the proverb "A rolling stone gathers no moss" as "Rolling stone, rolling stone, moss is green." Given this observation, most reviewers would suspect the validity of any further clinical information the psychiatrist recorded in the patients' medical charts.

In another instance, a therapist used exactly the same clinical note, with the patient's name and date changed, for several patients, hospitalized months apart. The ruse was detected when several medical records from the facility were examined by the same reviewer. Why would a practitioner perpetrate such a fraud, given the risk of detection and severe repercussions? Perhaps he assumed that he was safe, that no one would examine several of his cases at the same time. Perhaps he justified the practice by arguing that it would permit him to devote more time to patient care. Whatever his reasons, his action demonstrated a cynical belief that the clinical details of the patient's case were irrelevant, that the medical record was useless, and that his observations would have little if any impact on the manner in which other members of the treatment team provided care. Seeing this repetition of a clinical note, a reviewer would rightly question the appropriateness and quality of care delivered by the provider, the facility, and the facility's staff.

Sometimes stock phrases provide a clue to the standards of practice of a particular facility or clinical service. Several years ago, I worked in an institution struggling to maintain its fiscal stability. The chairman declared that in order to collect the maximum insurance payments for psychiatric services, a staff physician would have to see each inpatient and write a note in the patient's medical chart each weekend day and holiday. Staff members who did not comply were fined a sum of money equal to the amount that would have been collected from the insurance companies. This policy might have made some sense if the patients were being seen by psychiatrists who normally worked on the inpatient services. Unfortunately, most of the physicians making weekend rounds worked on other clinical services. Because they did not know the patients, they wrote a few bland phrases: "Patient seen. No complaints. Remains stable. Continue with current treatment." Like graffiti artists, they were documenting their presence for all to see, and nothing more.

The use of such stock, often meaningless, clinical phrases has not gone unnoticed by the health insurance industry. Its response has been to stipulate the specific details that must be included in each note if the practitioner and facility are to receive reimbursement for the treatment they provide.

These rules, enforced by the reviewer, demand that the practitioner state the content of the discussion with the patient, the specific treatment rendered, the patient's response, and the benefit the patient received. This is obviously an overreaction based on a mutual lack of trust. The problem will continue to escalate until the various sides arrive at an agreement that recognizes the practitioner's demand for a reasonable reimbursement and the insurance company's need for evidence that care has been provided according to expected standards.

Standardized Forms, Checklists, and Boilerplates

Some health care facilities openly endorse the use of stock phrases in clinical documentation, by establishing the practice as an institutional policy. Rather than developing individualized treatment plans for patients, they standardize their documentation to the point that it contains only boilerplate statements describing the general contents of the services provided. There is little if any documentation of the individual patient's clinical needs or treatment goals. Sometimes the goals are so nonspecific that they would sound foolish to the layperson. The treatment plan for each patient in a large community hospital demonstrates the problem. It stated, in part: "Goal 1: The patient will continue to feel well." Why would a facility include such a goal in its treatment plans? It is so generic that it is meaningless. Is not the goal of all treatment to help the patient remain (or become) well? In addition to being meaningless, the statement suggests that the patient has some control over whether he or she continues to feel well. Would any clinician write such a goal in the record of a patient with cancer or heart disease? Probably not. How then can it be used for a mental health disorder? Reviewers who see such goals tend to ignore them and to search for evidence that the staff have some definite objectives for the patient's treatment.

Standardized treatment plans are a particularly common problem in substance abuse rehabilitation programs that offer the same treatment program to every patient. In one such program, the standardization went so far that every patient had virtually identical progress notes and discharge summaries. The summaries contained a series of generic statements about the patient's progress, such as "He began to understand the reasons why he used abused substances" and "He committed himself to abstinence." When I asked the senior staff members of the facility how they could justify this policy, they defended it vigorously, stating that it was the only way they could efficiently treat patients in the allotted time. Moreover, they insisted that the policy represented a perfectly reasonable standard of care, one they would not change. They did not seem to understand that they were doing themselves and their patients a disservice with the policy. The major function of the medical record was nullified because the stock phrases did little to communicate the details of the patient's clinical condition to members of the current treatment team or subsequent therapists so that they could coordinate their care. Furthermore, even if the staff were providing the best clinical care possible, no reviewer would ever be able to verify this by reading the clinical documentation in the patients' medical charts.

Sometimes facilities adopt standardized report forms in a misguided attempt to improve quality of care. A few years ago, I was on the faculty of a large academic hospital. The nursing department, concerned that the documentation of care by individual nurses was not consistent, spent many months developing a three-page foldout form that was to be completed for every patient at the end of each shift. Because the form was to be used on every clinical service, much of the information requested tended to be irrelevant. This was particularly true in the case of patients on the psychiatric service. Nevertheless, the nursing staff completed the forms as best they could. As a result, the medical records were quickly filled with 20 or 30 forms or more, each with a few lines of information. The forms were so cumbersome that there was no easy way to follow the patient's progress over time. As a result, most clinicians completely ignored the forms. It would have been far better if the nursing staff had continued to record observations in linear sequence in the patient's record, as the other clinicians did.

Many health care facilities develop elaborate checklists for recording patients' signs, symptoms, behavior, and activities. Checklists must be differentiated from validated clinical scales. The latter are standardized methods of evaluating patients. Checklists are usually developed by individual practitioners or facilities and are means of recording the presence or absence of clinical information. Mental status examination findings are often recorded using checklists. The problem with many clinical checklists is that they do not satisfactorily convey the information they intend to convey, because they force practitioners to select answers that do not quite match the clinical phenomena they are observing. In addition, checklists are usually difficult to read and take up far more space than a simple narrative description. For those reasons, most reviewers ignore checklists. The only time they pay attention to them is when there is some inconsistency in the checklist that they can use to support their arguments and decisions.

Checklists can produce more problems for the facility than they solve because staff members rarely complete checklists in a consistent fashion.

This is especially true if the facility uses a series of checklists to follow a patient's progress over time. That problem was evident in one facility that used a checklist to document each patient's suicidal ideation and intent at the end of each nursing shift. In one particular case, the nurses on the first four shifts indicated on the checklist that the patient did have suicidal ideation and intent. Subsequent shifts, however, left that portion of the checklist blank. The medical director of the facility did not seem to be aware that the inconsistent use of the checklist made it look as if his clinical staff were not paying attention to the patient's symptoms and treatment. If a facility establishes a checklist to monitor a patient's clinical status, the staff must complete the checklist in a consistent manner. The more detailed the checklist, the less likely it is that this will happen.

Fortunately, few practitioners and facilities are as extreme in their use of generic documentation and forms as those I described. Yet too many seem unable to identify or communicate the clinical information that clearly differentiates one patient and his or her problems from another. There is simply no substitute for appropriate individualized documentation that clearly describes the patient and his or her clinical problems, treatment, and response to treatment. Your notes need not be extensive—merely pertinent to your patient's specific illness. Instead of rote statements such as "Insight-oriented and cognitive-behavioral therapy were provided to the patient in daily individual therapy sessions," consider this: "The patient learned, in cognitive therapy, to recognize the connection between negative thoughts about himself and the urge to drink." Instead of writing "The patient discussed family problems and learned how to respond more effectively to these problems," write: "The patient reported how intimidated and helpless he felt in arguments with his mother and learned techniques to respond more effectively to her and protect his self-esteem." To a reviewer, the second note of each pair provides far more convincing evidence of appropriate treatment than does the first, because it identifies the patient's unique problems and shows how you and the staff responded to them.

Clinical forms and checklists can be useful. Some facilities have developed forms that are convenient and collect standardized data yet still allow practitioners to enter individualized patient information. The secret is to be modest in your expectations rather than overinclusive. Do not try to develop a comprehensive form that collects every conceivable bit of clinical information. Do not try to anticipate all the possible answers to every question. Focus on the most important information. Use the form to guide practitioners in providing consistent information that is directly relevant to the patient's treatment. The most useful forms I have seen combine a specific symptom checklist with room for narrative reports. This can be done in surprisingly little space if the staff are trained to write succinct yet meaningful descriptions of the patient's clinical status, treatment, and response to treatment. The best example of this I have ever seen was a single-page form that had room, on one side, for three nursing shifts to report on the patient. The presence or absence of important mental status items (for example, suicidal ideation, agitation, confusion, or hallucinations) could be noted on a checklist for each shift. There was room under the checklist for the nurse to add a few lines of narrative about the patient. Anyone examining the chart—reviewer or clinician—could easily follow the patient's treatment and response to treatment over succeeding days. The Bauhaus maxim "Less is more" immediately came to mind as I read these forms. They told me exactly what I needed to know about the patient, and nothing more.

Write Detailed Yet Succinct Notes

In "Standardized Forms, Checklists, and Boilerplates," I argued that your clinical documentation should contain an individualized description of the patient's illness and progress in treatment, rather than a set of generic statements that are interchangeable from one patient to another. The judicious choice of pertinent clinical details is what individualizes a clinical note and makes it relevant. After reading such a note, another clinician should have a workable mental image of the patient and his or her problems.

You also have an obligation to be succinct, to make your notes cogent and readable, and to protect your patient's privacy. This may seem like a contradiction, but it is more a matter of balance and proportion. Some gifted practitioners have an uncanny ability to write a clinical note that focuses precisely on the most important issues in the patient's treatment. Most clinicians struggle to sharpen their focus to adequately describe the patient's condition and the treatment in the most succinct manner possible. I have reviewed thousands of medical records and observed a wide variation with respect to length and relevance of progress notes. At one extreme is the psychiatrist whose notes consist of "Patient doing better," "Patient less depressed," or "More upset today." At the other extreme is the psychiatrist who dictates two typed pages as each of his progress notes. The notes of the former communicate so little specific information that they could be applied to half the patients in the hospital. The notes of the latter are so contradictory and redundant, so filled with irrelevant material about the patient's family and how the family reacted to talking to the psychiatrist, that it is difficult to obtain any clear idea of the patient's condition or response to treatment. The reader is left with a sense that the psychiatrist has little idea what he or she is trying to do with the patient.

Clinical details are just as important in the written documentation as they are in the oral presentation to a reviewer. One common problem in many medical records is that clinical conclusions are stated without the necessary evidence to support them. It is not sufficient to report that a patient is agitated, psychotic, or manic; you must supply examples that demonstrate how these states are manifested by the patient and how they affect the patient's day-to-day functioning. If, for example, you state that the patient is having an acute psychotic episode, you must provide some of the details of that episode to make it come alive to the reader. If the patient wanders aimlessly around the hall, bangs his head against the wall when he's not in restraints, screams, yells, and assaults other patients, these symptoms should be described in the medical record. The reviewer is much more likely to approve your request for clinical care if he or she has enough clinical details to form a realistic image of the patient that is consistent with your assessment. If you are concerned that the patient is a danger to himself, document the detailed clinical observations that led you to that conclusion.

Remember that clinicians differ in what they consider conclusive clinical evidence. You might, for example, conclude that a patient is acutely suicidal because she states, "I can't go on like this any longer." Yet this statement could be interpreted in a number of different ways. The patient might be stating that she cannot go on working as hard as she has in the past. She might also mean that she cannot sleep as much or have as much sex as in the past. The only way to clarify what she means is to ask her, "What do you mean when you say 'I can't go on like this any longer?'" Yet many times such statements are interpreted to fit a clinician's picture of the patient's condition, without further verification from the patient. Worse, when asked to provide evidence to support their conclusions, some clinicians become indignant that their clinical judgment is being questioned. Often that anger stems from the embarrassing realization that they do not have any further detailed information about the patient's clinical condition.

It is trite to say that relevant information is important at every level of clinical decision making. Yet even the best physicians make decisions about their patients' care without clearly explaining the basis for their decisions. I was struck by this fact while reviewing the long-term treatment of a group of psychiatric outpatients who were prescribed antidepressant medications to treat their major depressive disorder. In the course of a year, many of the patients were prescribed several different antidepressant medications. In many of these cases, there was little documentation in the patient's medical record explaining why the physician decided to change the medications. The physicians were not providing poor care or trying to be evasive; they simply did not think it was necessary to explain the basis for their decisions. Unfortunately, the next physician who treats the patient will not know why he or she was switched from one medication to another. Did the medication have unacceptable side effects, was it ineffective, was it too costly? Each of these reasons has different implications for subsequent treatment. If, for example, the initial medication was very effective but was too costly, the next physician might be able to persuade the pharmaceutical company to provide the medication to the patient for free through its compassionate treatment program. That is one reason it is important to explain why you decide to start or discontinue treatment with a medication or change the dose of a medication. The note can be as simple as "The patient reported that she could not reach orgasm while taking sertraline" or "The patient has been taking fluoxetine 60 mg qd for 5 weeks without a decrease in her depression or insomnia."

One of the most common reasons for admitting a patient to the hospital is concern that the patient has suicidal ideation or intent. That particular clinical problem provides a useful lesson on the importance of detailed clinical information in the decision to approve or not approve a patient's admission. Consider the following hypothetical note by a psychiatrist seeking to admit a patient to the hospital:

> The patient is a 37-year-old businessman who has been depressed for a few months. His main complaint is a feeling of depression and difficulty making decisions. I've treated him with antidepressant medication in the last 2 months but he hasn't responded. The patient has a successful business and a supportive wife who is worried about him and is willing to do whatever she can to help him. His wife and I have finally convinced him that he needs to come into the hospital for further treatment.

Although the psychiatrist may have convinced his patient to be hospitalized, this note is unlikely to convince the reviewer that the patient requires hospitalization. Despite all his words, the psychiatrist has provided few relevant clinical details. His presentation would have been more convincing had he written this instead:

> The patient is a 37-year-old successful businessman who is severely depressed, with early morning awakening, moderate psychomotor retardation, a profound feeling of worthlessness, recurrent thoughts about dying, and growing indecisiveness that has significantly interfered with his ability to function at work. He has not responded to a combination of 60 mg of

fluoxetine and 150 mg of venlafaxine over the last month. I will treat him with electroconvulsive therapy (ECT). If he responds, I will continue the ECT on an outpatient basis.

The difference between the two notes lies in the clinical details provided. The second note, although a few words shorter than the first, describes the patient's clinical symptoms in enough detail for the reviewer to see that the diagnostic criteria for a DSM-IV-TR diagnosis of major depressive disorder have been met. It tells exactly how the psychiatrist has treated the patient, the outcome of that treatment, and his plan for further treatment in the hospital.

Be realistic. Even though you may be an experienced clinician, a reviewer cannot simply accept your credentials and experience as justification for your statements and decisions; corroborating evidence is needed. Place yourself in the reviewer's position and consider how you would react if you were forced to make a decision about a case on the basis of a few sparse comments by a physician whom you did not know. The likelihood is that you would feel very uncomfortable doing so without further evidence. Remember, reviewers increasingly have to be able to justify their decisions in the same way that you do. Therefore, if you state that a patient is still "suicidal" or "violent," the reviewer will want to read the evidence you used to reach this conclusion. You must support your opinion with relevant and pertinent observations of the patient's behavior and statements. If, for example, the patient became enraged at another patient the night before and began screaming at him and threatening him, you could cite this observation as evidence that the patient had not gained sufficient control of his behavior to be safely discharged. On the other hand, the fact that the patient got into an argument with a staff member is not convincing evidence that he is potentially violent. Do not even bother writing that a patient still has "the potential to be suicidal" or, as one uncertain practitioner wrote, "remains at risk for potential suicidal ideation." These statements are so speculative that they will do little to convince any clinician, let alone a skeptical reviewer, that a patient needs further hospitalization.

Writing a good clinical note is an active, not passive, process. The secret is to conceptualize the case, as I stated earlier—that is, to decide in advance what you need to say before you start writing. This is one of the hardest things to master in clinical practice. Remember, your notes in the medical record are the documentation of how you think about the patient's illness and treatment. You must discuss what matters clinically—what is necessary to satisfy the diagnostic criteria and treatment guidelines. Avoid cluttering your notes with gratuitous comments that are inconsistent with the patient's psychiatric disorder. Do not make the mistake of one practitioner, who wrote in the record of an agitated, aggressive patient with a bipolar disorder: "I told him to follow the Golden Rule in all his actions." Although the Golden Rule is a laudable moral precept, it is irrelevant advice for a patient whose psychiatric disorder precludes following it. Furthermore, the statement calls into question the practitioner's clinical management of the patient's case.

Reviewers generally do not believe that every bit of information about a patient is equally important for his or her treatment. Instead, they work with a subset of the clinical information collected by the practitioner. They focus on the current episode of illness and its immediate precipitants, on the patient's current symptoms, on the proposed date of discharge, and on the immediate follow-up plans. Although it is true that episodes of illness often have several contributing factors, most reviewers believe that a rule of diminishing returns, with respect to the amount of relevant information collected, applies in almost all of these cases. By that I mean that although some aspects of a patient's life contribute to his or her current illness, not everything does. When a patient with a bipolar disorder stops taking his lithium or sodium valproate, that single fact is much more important to the reviewer than the patient's educational history, his early developmental history, or his relationship with his siblings, unless you can clearly demonstrate that his noncompliance was directly related to these aspects of his life. This does not mean that you should stop documenting what you think is clinically relevant. It does mean that you should be sure to include the information that the reviewer needs if you want the case approved.

When you write something about a patient, you should be guided by a single precept: write only detailed information that is directly relevant to the patient's illness and treatment. This means, for example, that if the patient is having an affair with her boss's husband, you need not, and should not, identify the lover in the patient's medical record. It is sufficient to note that the patient is struggling with a problematic relationship with a man. To write more details about this relationship may betray the patient's confidence and perhaps subject her to unnecessary pain and suffering. No reviewer will care about the identity of the patient's lover, and no one else who has access to the record needs to know the identity. Anyone who treats the patient will quickly discover the nature of the relationship during therapy.

I learned this lesson the hard way many years ago, while still in training. I had been treating a young woman with a severe personality disorder (most probably borderline personality disorder) who frequently regressed to an infantile state in which she communicated in baby talk and cut herself to relieve her intense anxiety. After 2 years of treatment, she was doing marginally better and decided to move to another city. I offered to refer her to a new psychiatrist, but she refused my offer, explaining that she would find a therapist for herself.

Several weeks later, I received a letter from a therapist asking for information about my former patient's treatment. He enclosed a release of information form signed by the patient. I responded with a detailed letter describing her diagnosis and treatment. Had I stopped there, I would have appropriately discharged my duty to the patient. Unfortunately, I added a few gratuitous comments about her inability to form stable relationships with men and the unlikelihood that she would be able to do so in the near future. A week later, I received a blistering letter from the patient, rightfully excoriating me for my casual, and insensitive, predictions about her prognosis. Her new therapist had, for whatever reasons, given her my letter. In a few irrelevant lines, I had endangered the modest gains made in 2 years of treatment. This incident taught me to ask myself the following question before writing anything about a patient: Is this information crucial for the patient's treatment and does it have the potential to compromise or harm the patient?

Suggested Reading

Baker JG, Shanfeld SB, Schnee S: Using quality improvement teams to improve documentation in records at a community mental health center. Psychiatr Serv 51:239–242, 2000

Tang PC, LaRosa MP, Gorden SM: Use of computer-based records, completeness of documentation, and appropriateness of documented clinical decisions. J Am Med Inform Assoc 6:245–251, 1999

Index

*Page numbers printed in **boldface** refer to tables or figures.*